Women & Health

This book delves into the critical issue of cancer as one of the leading causes of death for women across diverse backgrounds, highlighting the alarming racial disparities across healthcare for women that affect mortality rates for Black, Indigenous, and Women of Color.

Though heart disease is the number one (21.8%) leading cause of death for females of all races, origins, and ages, cancer is a close second at 20.7%. The experiences of women in cancer range across identities and the systems in which they exist. Cancer does not only impact the diagnosed, but all those around them. This volume provides a wealth of information for consideration for both mental health and medical professionals.

This book is an invaluable resource for students and researchers in mental health and psychology, as well as healthcare providers and policymakers interested in public health, women's studies, and healthcare.

The chapters in this book were originally published in the *Journal of Feminist Family Therapy*.

Kristina S. Brown is Professor and the Chair of the Couple and Family Therapy at Adler University. She is the Editor-in-Chief of the *Journal of Feminist Family Therapy* and Editor of the new *AAMFT Systemic Ethics Textbook*. Dr. Brown is a feminist qualitative researcher with a broad focus on the experiences of women across identities as represented in her scholarly work. She lives in her "empty nest" in the Chicago Loop with her husband of 30 years and their two polydactyl cats, Cameron and Ferris.

Feminist Family Therapy

The books in this series delve into the intersections of gender, power, and culture, providing innovative therapeutic approaches that challenge traditional narratives. The *Feminist Family Therapy* book series contains a wide range of the journal's special issues and features contributions from leading experts in the field. The series addresses diverse family structures and experiences, promoting empowerment and social justice. The books in this series are ideal for practitioners, scholars, and students and they serve as essential resources for anyone seeking to understand and transform the complexities of family life in modern society.

Recent books in the series include

Women's Reproductive and Sexual Health
Edited by Kristina Brown

Women's Health
Gender and Pain
Edited by Kristina Brown

Women & Health
Women and Cancer
Edited by Kristina Brown

Women & Health
Women and Cancer

**Edited by
Kristina S. Brown**

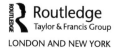

LONDON AND NEW YORK

First published 2025
by Routledge
4 Park Square, Milton Park, Abingdon, Oxon, OX14 4RN

and by Routledge
605 Third Avenue, New York, NY 10158

Routledge is an imprint of the Taylor & Francis Group, an informa business

© 2025 Taylor & Francis

All rights reserved. No part of this book may be reprinted or reproduced or utilised in any form or by any electronic, mechanical, or other means, now known or hereafter invented, including photocopying and recording, or in any information storage or retrieval system, without permission in writing from the publishers.

Trademark notice: Product or corporate names may be trademarks or registered trademarks, and are used only for identification and explanation without intent to infringe.

British Library Cataloguing in Publication Data
A catalogue record for this book is available from the British Library

ISBN13: 978-1-032-71839-2 (hbk)
ISBN13: 978-1-032-71841-5 (pbk)
ISBN13: 978-1-032-71842-2 (ebk)

DOI: 10.4324/9781032718422

Typeset in Minion Pro
by Newgen Publishing UK

Publisher's Note
The publisher accepts responsibility for any inconsistencies that may have arisen during the conversion of this book from journal articles to book chapters, namely the inclusion of journal terminology.

Disclaimer
Every effort has been made to contact copyright holders for their permission to reprint material in this book. The publishers would be grateful to hear from any copyright holder who is not here acknowledged and will undertake to rectify any errors or omissions in future editions of this book.

Contents

Citation Information vi
Notes on Contributors viii

Introduction: Women and Cancer 1
Kristina S. Brown

1 Diagnosis, Prognosis and Caregiving: An Autoethnography 3
Karen Parker

2 Breast Cancer and Body Image: Feminist Therapy Principles and Interventions 20
Chiquita Holmes, Alexis Jackson, Joan Looby, Kasia Gallo, and Kendra Blakely

3 Therapeutic Interventions with Families of Breast Cancer Survivors 40
Alexis Jackson, Chiquita Holmes, Joan Looby, and Kendra Blakely

4 Relationship of Optimism, Pessimism, and Dysfunctional Career Thoughts in Breast Cancer Survivors from the Bahamas 59
Levette S. Scott, Carlos P. Zalaquett, Herbert Exum, Jeffrey D. Kromrey, Cheryl R. Ellerbrock, and Raheem J. Paxton

5 Gender Roles and the Family Life Cycle: The Case of Women with Cancer 81
Larra Petersen, Theresa Kruczek and Angela Shaffner

6 Feminist-Informed Medical Family Therapy Principles and Techniques Across Biopsychosocial Systems Levels for Younger Women with Breast Cancer and Their Partners 98
Stephanie R. Burwell, Bowden Templeton, Kelly S. Kennedy and Lisa Zak-Hunter

Index 119

Citation Information

The chapters in this book were originally published in the *Journal of Feminist Family Therapy*, volume 33, issue 1 (2021), except Chapters 5 and 6, which were published in volume 15, issue 2-3 (2004), and volume 20, issue 2 (2008). When citing this material, please use the original page numbering for each article, as follows:

Introduction
Women and Cancer
Kristina S. Brown
Journal of Feminist Family Therapy, volume 33, issue 1 (2021), pp. 1–2

Chapter 1
Diagnosis, Prognosis and Caregiving: An Autoethnography
Karen Parker
Journal of Feminist Family Therapy, volume 33, issue 1 (2021), pp. 3–19

Chapter 2
Breast Cancer and Body Image: Feminist Therapy Principles and Interventions
Chiquita Holmes, Alexis Jackson, Joan Looby, Kasia Gallo, and Kendra Blakely
Journal of Feminist Family Therapy, volume 33, issue 1 (2021), pp. 20–39

Chapter 3
Therapeutic Interventions with Families of Breast Cancer Survivors
Alexis Jackson, Chiquita Holmes, Joan Looby, and Kendra Blakely
Journal of Feminist Family Therapy, volume 33, issue 1 (2021), pp. 40–58

Chapter 4
Relationship of Optimism, Pessimism, and Dysfunctional Career Thoughts in Breast Cancer Survivors from the Bahamas
Levette S Scott, Carlos P Zalaquett, Herbert Exum, Jeffrey D Kromrey, Cheryl R Ellerbrock, and Raheem J. Paxton
Journal of Feminist Family Therapy, volume 33, issue 1 (2021), pp. 59–80

Chapter 5
Gender Roles and the Family Life Cycle: The Case of Women with Cancer
Larra Petersen, Theresa Kruczek and Angela Shaffner
Journal of Feminist Family Therapy, volume 15, issue 2-3 (2004), pp. 99–119

Chapter 6
Feminist-Informed Medical Family Therapy Principles and Techniques Across Biopsychosocial Systems Levels for Younger Women with Breast Cancer and Their Partners
Stephanie R. Burwell, Bowden Templeton, Kelly S. Kennedy and Lisa Zak-Hunter
Journal of Feminist Family Therapy, volume 20, issue 2 (2008), pp. 99–125

For any permission-related enquiries please visit:
www.tandfonline.com/page/help/permissions

Notes on Contributors

Kendra Blakely, Department of Counseling, Educational Psychology & Foundations, Mississippi State University, Starkville, Mississippi, USA.

Kristina S. Brown, Couple and Family Therapy, Adler University, Chicago, Illinois, USA.

Stephanie R. Burwell, Department of Child and Family Development, University of Georgia, Georgia, USA.

Cheryl R. Ellerbrock, University of South Florida, Florida, USA.

Herbert Exum, University of South Florida, Florida, USA.

Kasia Gallo, Department of Counseling, Educational Psychology & Foundations, Mississippi State University, Starkville, Mississippi, USA.

Chiquita Holmes, Department of Counseling, Educational Psychology & Foundations, Mississippi State University, Starkville, Mississippi, USA.

Alexis Jackson, Department of Counseling, Educational Psychology & Foundations, Mississippi State University, Starkville, Mississippi, USA.

Kelly S. Kennedy, Department of Child and Family Development, University of Georgia, Georgia, USA.

Jeffrey D. Kromrey, University of South Florida, Florida, USA.

Theresa Kruczek, Counseling Psychology Program, Ball State University, Muncie, Indiana, USA.

Joan Looby, Department of Counseling, Educational Psychology & Foundations, Mississippi State University, Starkville, Mississippi, USA.

Karen Parker, College of Arts, Sciences and Education, Texas A&M University, Texarkana, Texas, USA.

Raheem J. Paxton, University of Alabama, Alabama, USA.

Larra Petersen, Counseling Psychology, Ball State University, Muncie, Indiana, USA; Cancer Center, Ball Memorial Hospital, Muncie, Indiana, USA.

Levette S. Scott, North Carolina Central University, North Carolina, USA.

Angela Shaffner, Counseling Psychology Program, Ball State University, Muncie, Indiana, USA.

Bowden Templeton, University of Georgia, Georgia, USA; Mercer University School of Medicine, Macon, Georgia, USA.

Lisa Zak-Hunter, Department of Child and Family Development, University of Georgia, Georgia, USA.

Carlos P. Zalaquett, Penn State University, Pennsylvania, USA.

Introduction: Women and Cancer

Kristina S. Brown

Though heart disease is the number one (21.8%) leading cause of death for females of all races, origins, and ages, cancer is a close second at 20.7% (CDC, https://www.cdc.gov/women/lcod/2017/all-races-origins/index.htm). Further, the racial disparities across healthcare for women further increases the mortality rates for Black, Indigenous, and Women of Color. This final and fifth issue of articles on women's health as part of a special call for submissions focuses on cancer.

In *Diagnosis, Prognosis and Caregiving: An Autoethnography*, our anonymous author shares a powerful firsthand experience of caregiving for her wife who was diagnosed with terminal endometrial cancer. Utilizing art – which is included throughout the article – as well as their experience as a lesbian couple navigating the healthcare system. Our second and third articles are *Breast Cancer and Body Image: Feminist Therapy Principles and Interventions, Part I* by Chiquita Holmes, Alexis Jackson, Joan Looby, Kasia Gallo, and Kendra Blakely and *Therapeutic Interventions with Families of Breast Cancer Survivors, Part II* by Alexis Jackson, Chiquita Holmes, Joan Looby, and Kendra Blakely. In the first article, the authors specifically look at body image and breast cancer especially from the experiences of women of color and lesbians. The second part presents specifical interventions that can be used therapeutically with families to support the member with breast cancer. Authors Levette Scott, Carlos P. Zalaquett, Herbert Exum, Jeffrey D. Kromrey, Cheryl R. Ellerbrock, and Raheem J. Paxton looked at the *Relationship of Optimism, Pessimism, and Dysfunctional Career Thoughts in Breast Cancer Survivors from the Bahamas* with the goal of assisting survivors with the multiple levels of impact of breast cancer.

Included in this book are also two earlier articles focusing on the experiences of cancer. Larra Petersen, Theresa Kurczek, and Angela Shaffer looked at *Gender Roles and the Family Life Cycle: The Case of Women with Cancer*. Centering a case student of a woman with breast cancer, the authors explored the intersection of the systemic experience of cancer with gender-role socialization, family systems and the family life cycle.

The final chapter by Stephanie R. Bruwell, Bowden Templeton, Kelly S. Kennedy, and Lisa Zak-Hunter, *Feminist-Informed Medical Family Therapy Principles and Techniques Across Biopsychosocial Systems Levels for Younger*

Women with Breast Cancer and their Partners, focused on the experiences of younger women (aged 50 and under). The authors present an integrated feminist-informed medical family therapy model to implement in supporting patients and their partners through the phases of cancer.

Diagnosis, Prognosis and Caregiving: An Autoethnography

Karen Parker

ABSTRACT
In this article, the complexity of the grieving process of the caregiver and her partner is discussed. Through an autoethnography, the author gives a voice to her personal story about her wife's diagnosis of endometrial cancer, her prognosis and the specialized considerations of a lesbian couple in the health care system. In order to understand the experiences of a lesbian couple's journey while interacting with the health care system, this autoethnography was written from a first-person perspective. Through the use of art, journal entries, and bicycle riding to navigate this journey, this unique study expands the conversation to include a systemic understanding of the effects of terminal illnesses on intimate relationships.

Introduction

Sometimes, when a person is diagnosed with cancer, the diagnosis becomes a part of every relationship that person has, especially intimate ones. All the person's conversations, schedules, daily routines become about cancer. Because there are specialized considerations in lesbians' relationships with the healthcare system (Hirsch et al., 2016), I decided to write an autoethnography from the context of a lesbian couple, in the southeastern region of the United States, relating to the healthcare system.

An autoethnography is, but not limited to, a form of qualitative research in which an author uses self-reflection and narrative writing to explore personal experience and connect this autobiographical story to a wider cultural understanding (Creswell & Poth, 2017; Ellis & Bochner, 2000). Autoethnographies are positioned as ethnographic inquiries using the researcher's autobiographical materials as primary data (Chang, 2008). Because traditional forms of ethnography do not value how connected a researcher's life experiences are to a broader culture (Mizzi, 2010), this autoethnography is presented including journal entries and paintings about my lived experiences as well as sharing my love of riding my bicycle.

Although some scholars deny the space that art belongs in research, others have attempted to explain how art and research intersect (Williams, 2009). Sullivan (2008) posits that art is research and states:

> The study of painting as an inquiry process that takes into account more than the physical and formal practices of creating images on surfaces. Not only is the artist involved in a 'doing' performance, but this also results in an image that is a site for further interpretation by viewers and an object that is part of a visual culture. (pp. 240-241)

Although I consider the artwork in this article as a part of the process of writing this autoethnography, I also considered my act of painting as therapeutic. Sometimes, when discussing my wife's illness became emotionally overwhelming, I would paint. The act of painting gave me a tool in which to articulate emotions that were overwhelming for me.

This study has two purposes: to illustrate how my relationship with art helped me through the process of caring for my wife and helping her navigate living with cancer, and to examine how my painting helped guide my journey. I also hope this autoethnography adds to the literature that shows how complicated grief and loss can be in lesbian couples and the positive impact that art can have on this pain experience. Because some lesbians have had significant losses due to homophobic family, friends and coworkers, when they lose an intimate partner, they may be losing a tremendous part of their emotional support system and social circle. Some lesbians have rejection as part of their lived experiences, and this could influence the way they interpret the world around them (Bauer & Bonanno, 2001; Davis & Nolen-Hoeksema, 2001). Art has always guided my interpretation of the world around me and has helped me cope with some of the most difficult events in my life.

Writing, riding, and painting the story into existence

Writing about writing

For me, writing is a process and writing an autoethnography is a journey that requires delving into emotions that are uncomfortable. I decided to begin by writing about writing, so the story itself would form the tones of the voices involved. To set the foundation, I am sharing my writing that began the development of this article. On this day, I was extremely sad, and my mind felt chaotic. To make sense of the chaos, I wrote this journal entry:

> I sit with literature in front of me to process through my feelings. I am unbelievably lonely right now. I know that my wife is experiencing cancer and chemotherapy and illness and fear. I feel immobilized by my fear of losing someone I truly love. I have looked for some solace in the literature I have read, but it is somehow not enough. I want to be able to get my story on paper, in some logical form. I am in the middle of something I find terrifying and surreal. The only way my mind can handle everything, I must write,

paint and imagine that I have the energy to ride my bicycle. The pouring of my emotions onto a canvas and letting the paint spill the story onto the paper will help me imagine ever riding a bicycle again.

Writing about riding

One activity that reduces stress in my life is riding my beach cruiser. I love my beach cruiser, because it is a simple way of getting from one place to the other. It does not have gears or handlebar brakes. It is like the bicycles I had as a kid where you just made one backward motion on the pedal and you stop. Riding my bike feels free and takes me back to a place where I felt carefree. In this article, I chose to use the image of the bicycle to navigate the metaphor needed to tell our story.

According to Macy (2011), during the 1890's, bicycles made a huge impact on women's suffrage. During this time, the bicycle also influenced the way women dressed. In order to ride bicycles more comfortably, women changed from wearing dresses with tight waists, corsets and tight necklines to lighter skirts, bloomers, split skirts and sometimes pants. These changes in clothing and the accessibility to her own form of transportation revolutionized the women's movement. Because navigating through the process of grief is unique for each person, the image of the individuality and freedom that bicycles have afforded women is important to giving voice to my story. I am also using the metaphor of the bicycle to illustrate how, as a caregiver, I have had to adjust to relationship changes in response to a cancer diagnosis. My role in my relationship has gone through many changes, so I found it necessary to create an image of change by using the bicycle as my story-telling vehicle.

Writing about painting

In addition to using the metaphor of the bicycle to navigate our story, I also used art as an avenue for expression and self-care. Because our story is emotionally difficult to narrate, I chose to use paintings as a guide. As I painted each painting, it helped organize the narration and made meaning of my experiences as a caregiver. As Sullivan (2008) states, "Whether seen as a process or product, the practice of painting can be argued to be a robust form of human engagement that has the potential to reveal new insights and understandings" (pp. 241–242). I painted my experiences in black and white with one item in each painting having color. I did this because right now my life seems a bit black and white with grays hovering in the background. The color represents ... Because I am telling this story in the here and now, as well as, retrospectively, my paintings are helping me give order to the narrative.

While planning to write this autoethnography, I decided that my wife, Tammy's voice needed to be heard as well. I wanted to write this, discussing my caregiving and our relationship roles, but I realized that when people are diagnosed with cancer, it seems like their voices fade into the background, as decisions sometimes must be made for them. I asked Tammy, "Sweetheart, do you mind occasionally answering questions about our journey and do you mind if I discuss your answers and our conversations in my article?" To which she responded, "If I am not feeling sick when you ask the questions, I would be glad to answer those questions and I do not mind if you discuss my answers." With that conversation, I decided that the best way for the readers to hear Tammy's voice in my article was to include conversations that we have had over the past year.

Our story

A few months ago, Tammy and I went on a brief vacation. We decided that we wanted to spend some time together while Tammy had the energy to travel. It was the

first day of our vacation and I was excited that we were headed to the beach. We were going to Pass Christian, a small beach town in Mississippi, where we were going to ride our beach cruisers around the small quaint town and spend several hours a day on the beach. It was a typical get-ready-to-go morning, where my wife and I were loading our clothes, food and dogs for our excursion. At last, we loaded our bicycles on the bike rack. Although I had a "gut feeling" that I should secure my pink beach cruiser with more bungee cords, I ignored my intuition and thought to myself, "It will be fine. I am just a bit anxious about our trip and the bicycle did not budge when I tried to wiggle it." As we traveled along the interstate, our excitement grew, until suddenly, my wife looked in the rearview mirror and said, "We just lost your bike. It fell. I am so sorry, babe. Let's go back and see if we can save it." We pulled to the side of the interstate and began to back up until we got to where my bicycle had fallen. Just as we reached where my bike fell, a semitruck ran over my bicycle. After the truck passed us, Tammy ran out and dragged it to the side of the road. I said to her, "It is ok. I need a new bicycle anyway." We got back into our vehicle and began driving toward our destination and it suddenly hit me. I began to cry. I knew my crying was not about my bicycle. It was about the year that my wife and I had endured. I really needed to cry, and the loss of my bicycle gave me the opportunity to release my emotions.

A year before this trip, Tammy, was diagnosed with stage-four endometrial cancer. This was our first vacation since her diagnosis. We had been through one of the most difficult years of our lives. Tammy woke up one day with some pelvic pain and within a month she was diagnosed with cancer and not given a good prognosis. We found out she had a rare form of endometrial cancer called papillary serous carcinoma. After her diagnosis, I read every article I could find concerning her cancer. "Uterine papillary serous carcinoma (UPSC) is a distinct histologic type of endometrial cancer which is associated with a high relapse rate and poor prognosis" (Goff et al., 1994, p. 264). I found similar statements and definitions in every article I read. This was devastating, but reading article after article helped me read through the process of acceptance.

I have found comfort with Hall's (2014) explanation that more conventional grief models have been abandoned to embrace the uniqueness of individual experiences. He posits, "Any interventions must be tailored to the uniqueness of the person, relationship and circumstances that characterize a client at a particular point in time as they grieve a specific loss" (Hall, 2014, p. 12). Although I find comfort in Kübler-Ross's (1969) stages of grief, I also find that, because I am still in the process of taking care of my wife, my grief is extraordinarily complicated.

Endometrial cancer: diagnosis and prognosis

I first painted the little girl in the swing (Figure 1), because when Tammy was diagnosed with cancer, I felt like I was hanging in midair and nothing seemed real. During Tammy's first hospitalization, I would sometimes walk down the hall to the waiting room where there was glass, so one could see the lobby from the waiting room. We were on the third floor and I would watch as people entered the hospital, coming and going. It was like I was hanging there, watching people go on with their lives as if nothing was happening to mine. My world had changed overnight and I could not move. This painting somehow articulated my life in a way words could not. I was hanging midair, not moving and my swing had no tree to which to anchor. I felt alone and somewhat ashamed, because my life had not prepared me for what was happening to my wife and me.

In the beginning, I really had difficulty dealing with the amount of pain Tammy was experiencing. Because we do not live in a large city, it took about a month for her to see a surgeon and an oncologist. While we were waiting to see a surgeon and an oncologist, her pain grew increasingly worse and we ended up in the emergency room several times. During one of the two times Tammy was hospitalized, I begged the nurses to do something about her pain. They shook their heads and told me that the doctor (hospitalist) had to approve her pain medications. But the doctor said that I needed to take her home, because the insurance company was refusing to pay for her hospitalization. When he said this, Tammy looked at me and cried.

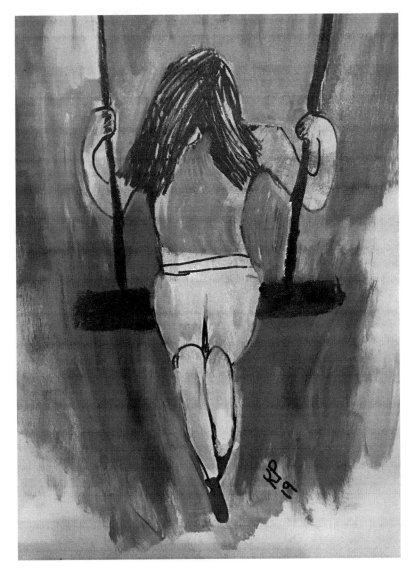

Figure 1. Diagnosis and prognosis.

During this first hospitalization, I also tried to be at the hospital every single time the doctor came into the room., but I found out that it was impossible, because I needed to shower, change clothes, eat and sometimes sleep. I was unbelievably stressed and devastated, so family members stayed at the hospital for me get to go home for a few minutes. During one of my trips to my house to check on our animals, shower and eat, one of the oncologists visited Tammy's hospital room. When I got back to the hospital and walked into her room and looked at Tammy's face, I could tell that something was terribly wrong. There were several family members in the room, so Tammy asked me to help her to the bathroom, and as she sat on the toilet, she buried her face into my abdomen and began to cry. She said through her tears, "It is not good, babe. I only have eighteen months to live." Like in my painting of the young girl in the swing (Figure 1), I felt suspended in surrealism. I stood there, but with all of the vocabulary in my arsenal, I didn't know what to say, so I said, "We have to have hope. Faith, hope and our love are all that we have." Later that night, while my wife was sleeping, I wrote the following journal entry:

> I cannot believe that my wife has eighteen months to live. I have no idea what to do. I act strong in front of her, but I AM NOT! I feel like raging because this is not fair. She is a good person. She is way better than I am. She loves life! She deserves to live more than I deserve to live! I love her and I do not want to lose her . . . .please GOD, tell me this is just a dream.

This hospitalization lasted a few more days and during this time, we finally saw an oncologist that told us he believed that he could get her pain under control with a combination of pain medication and chemotherapy. This doctor helped me manage her pain. He listened and slowly increased her pain medications. About six months later, after her chemotherapy began to work, a complete hysterectomy and the removal of the lining of her abdomen, her pain began to subside, and Tammy stopped taking pain medications.

Discrimination

Although Tammy was pain-free after several months, until then, we continued to fight the pain. I remember one night when Tammy had gone to bed in excruciating pain. She woke up about two o'clock in the morning, clinging to me, squeezing my hand and crying, so we headed to the emergency room. On this night, the nurse looked me up and down. Her eyes began at the top of my head and scanned down my body to my feet and then back up where they landed on my face. I will never forget the smirk on her face and the question that she asked me. She said, "And who are you?" To which I replied, "I am her wife and I have copies of our marriage license and my power of attorney, if you would like to see them." She shook her head and ignored me the rest of our visit. As I painted this person (Figure 2), who is hanging onto the handkerchief in her pocket, I thought of the discrimination that Tammy and I faced during her treatment. I thought of how thankful I was to have a marriage license and power of attorney to which I cling. I also painted this painting to help articulate the intense sadness I felt. Sometimes when I would take a walk away from my wife's hospital room, I would sit in the waiting room, crying and clinging to tissues I had in my pocket. Somehow, the soft texture of the tissues kept me centered enough to think about what I needed to do next to take care of my wife.

Although we have had to face subtle discrimination throughout her treatment, we also faced blatant discrimination. After months of chemotherapy,

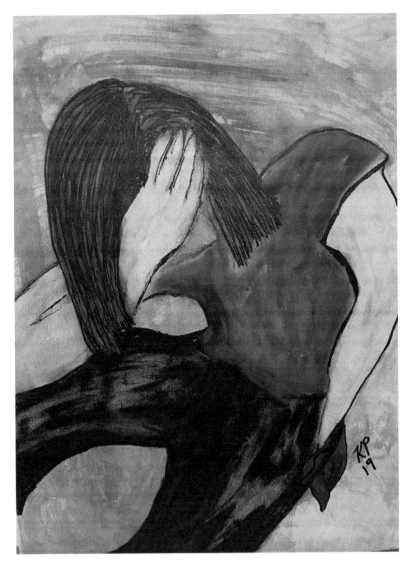

Figure 2. Discrimination.

Tammy had a hysterectomy which would also remove a large portion of her cancer. We knew that the surgeon would not be able to remove all of it, but this surgery would reduce the pain and hopefully increase her life expectancy. The morning of Tammy's hysterectomy, the nurse took her into the room where they started her IV and performed blood work on her. The nurse told me to have a seat in the waiting room and they would call me back when they had Tammy ready for surgery. The wait was unbearable. After an hour, I texted Tammy to see if they had mentioned me getting to see her before her surgery. Tammy texted back that she had asked but had gotten no response. I was very anxious and becoming more agitated, so I texted Tammy and asked if she would try one more time to get the nurse to let me see her before she went into surgery. The nurse finally came to the waiting room and took me to see her. Tammy then told me that when she buzzed the nurse and asked could her wife come back to see her, the nurse responded, "Your who?" Tammy responded, "Can my wife come back to see me now?" The nurse responded, "Don't you mean your family?" Tammy said, "No. I mean my wife." The nurse then said, "Okay. I will call for your family." They came to the waiting room and called for the family of Tammy Parker and I went back to see her before they rolled her down to the operating room. Because they were trying to remove as much of the cancer as possible, the surgery lasted four excruciating hours. Thankfully, Tammy made it through the surgery and came home the next day. I went home later that evening and I was relieved that I could vent the following in my journal:

> I am proud of myself, because I did not completely lose my mind with the hospital staff. It felt passive aggressive when they let me sit in the waiting room that long. When I found out about the way they treated Tammy when she asked for her wife. IT IS 2018 ... .please! They need to GROW UP! I am extremely scared for Tammy! The surgeon said that her cancer is "extensive." I am overwhelmed. It is very difficult to breathe. The amount of anxiety I have right now is overwhelming, but I am embarrassed about not being able to handle my anxiety. I am scared to talk to people about what I really feel.

I am very grateful that I can journal and paint my way through some of the discrimination. According to Fallin-Bennett (2015), there have been shifts in society's attitude toward the LGBTQ community. Explicit discrimination has become socially unacceptable, while implicit discrimination remains widespread. According to the 2019 Health Equality Index, 56% of LGBT people experience discrimination from the health care system. Because of the discrimination experienced by LGBT+ individuals, we search for providers who are comfortable with our affectional orientation (Neville & Henrickson, 2006).

Our relationship before and after the diagnosis

I chose to paint (Figure 3) two women dancing to represent my relationship with my wife before and after the diagnosis. I compare our relationship to a dance with moves, sways, and turns. Our relationship before the diagnosis was a great, a give-and-take dance. After the diagnosis, our relationship was still a dance, but that dance had a different rhythm. In the painting of the silhouette of the women, one is wearing a red dress. This represents the love Tammy and I have. This love has guided us through the dark times of this journey. It has been and is still difficult for both of us to "wrap our heads" around her diagnosis and prognosis. When I asked Tammy to describe our relationship before and after her diagnosis, her response was the following:

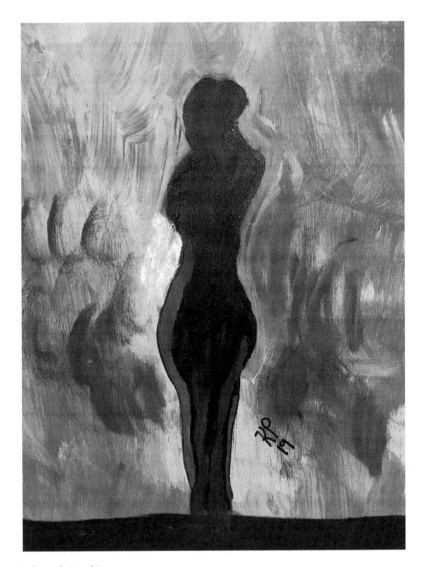

Figure 3. Our relationship.

> Well, before, it was more equal. I took care of the house and you did your part. We were also more active. Now, you have more responsibility. I think I rely on you a lot more and I know that puts a lot of pressure on you. I feel sad and guilty for putting you through this. I also feel frustrated that I cannot do the things I use to do. We are intimate, but not sexually intimate, because of the type cancer I have and the amount of pain I have experienced. It is just so sad to lose the life that we had. We are so compatible. Our life is still good. I am not saying that it is not good now. I am just saying it is so different.

I agree with Tammy on the changes in our relationship. When Tammy was first diagnosed, she was in a tremendous amount of pain. I remember when Tammy first came home from her first hospital stay, I had to check on her every thirty minutes and administer her medication every ninety minutes, twenty-four hours a day. Although I was still in shock and was very sad, I had to keep going! I had to set an alarm for every ninety minutes, so I could keep Tammy out of pain. I had to accept that our relationship had evolved from our being equals into a relationship where I was the caregiver. My role with my wife became more like a parent. I made sure she took her medication and nagged her about eating, so her body could endure the chemotherapy. One of the many adjustments I had to accept was the fact that Tammy was so heavily medicated and much of the time, she was not aware of my presence. Our lives suddenly revolved around pain management, chemotherapy, doctor's appointments, PET scans, hospitalizations, and my wife's wishes concerning her affairs.

Self-care

In the beginning, because of the extensive amount of pain medications and chemotherapy medications Tammy had to take, she was hot all the time and wanted the temperature in our house extremely low. Although it was almost one hundred degrees outside, inside our house, I would dress for the winter. One night, Tammy woke up, rolled over and said, "You look like a monk. Are you cold? You have a hoodie on in bed." I responded with, "Yeah. It is freezing in here." Before I finished my sentence, she had fallen back to sleep. The next morning, while sitting in our living room, I glanced out on the patio and saw colorful birds and green plants. Everything was alive out there. I got up from the couch, walked over to the French doors and opened them to find a spot on our side patio where I could sit. It was very warm out there and that, somehow, comforted me. I called this one patio chair my "cancer-free" zone.

My "cancer-free" zone is why I chose to paint a picture of a chair to depict one way I was able to take care of myself. (Figure 4) I had one place to rest my mind. I had to create this zone because, at first, I obsessed about Tammy's diagnosis. I began to have panic attacks and hide in the bathroom and practice relaxation techniques. I kept telling myself that I was a counselor and family therapist and should be able to manage my anxiety. When I found my place outside where I would allow myself not to think about cancer, I finally calmed my spirit. When I sat in my chair, I would watch nature, would stare at the green leaves of plants that Tammy has kept alive for years, and would watch birds fly into the feeders we have out there. For some reason this would nourish my resolve. I would meditate and pray. On the other hand, I would sometimes feel guilty that I had a place that I could pretend that cancer did not exist. I felt guilty, because Tammy had no place to escape.

Sometimes people say, "What can I do for you?" I never know what to say to them. It is difficult for me to tell someone what to do for me. I tell them to pray for me to know what to do for Tammy. I constantly wonder if I am doing enough or doing the right thing. I think self-care is extremely important when someone is caregiving a loved one. I have found that when people offer to

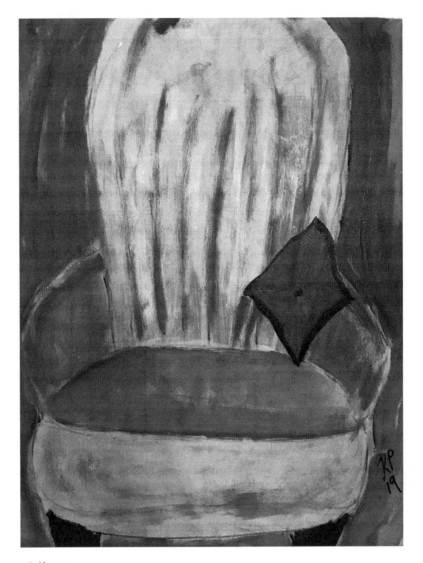

Figure 4. Self-care.

clean my house or cook for us, I let them. I am constantly having to let go of some of my perceived control over a situation that is not really in my control. I also spoke with my doctor about anti-anxiety medication. I began taking medication twice a day and my anxiety became controlled enough for me to cope. Taking care of myself is the key to my healing.

Forced to consider My Life without My Wife

A few weeks ago, we were sitting on our patio after Tammy found out the results of her most recent biopsy of her lymph nodes. The biopsy was positive for metastatic disease, which meant it was positive for cancer. We were both crying. It was the first time we had cried at the same time, but crying was the only place we could go. Tammy took my hands into both of her hands and said, "If you write this article about us, just let them know what we have gone through. Let them know how hard it is, how difficult it is not to know how much time I have. I don't know if it is months, weeks. I just don't know. Nobody knows."

I chose to paint a person under the umbrella to express how emotionally dark it was for me when I first heard Tammy's prognosis and had to consider my life without her (Figure 5). I think this painting was the most difficult for me to paint, because it is overwhelming. I painted the umbrella extremely large, because the weight of self-protection feels larger than I am. When I look

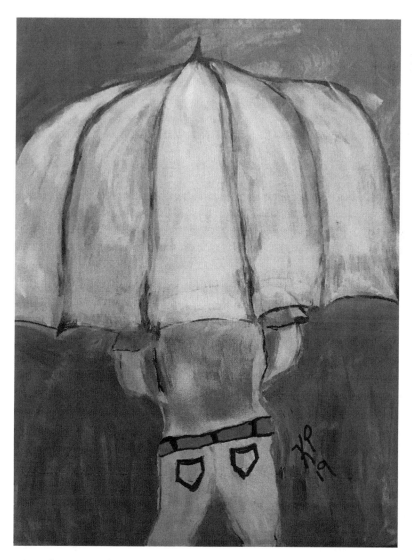

Figure 5. Considering My Life without My Wife.

at this painting, I feel the loss of "my place in the world." When I am with Tammy, I feel a sense of belonging, a sense of purpose. Even now, with all the caregiving that I do, I feel that caring for her is the single most important thing I have ever done.

Whenever I do think about my future without her, I feel a tremendous amount of guilt. I realized that much of our lives are spent looking forward to the future. We spend a lot of time thinking about what we are going to do next, what our careers are going to look like in five years, what we are going to do when we retire, etc. When my spouse was given a poor prognosis, thinking about the future became extremely sad and guilt-ridden for me. I journaled right after I painted the umbrella painting:

> When I look at this painting, I feel lonely. Although I came into my relationship with Tammy as an independent person, we learned to rely on each other. She taught me that I could let someone in, let them close to me, let them care for me without losing my independence. I had been in relationships before where the person would try to change me. Tammy has never tried to change me. She has just accepted and loved me. Although, thinking of my life without Tammy feels lonely, I am so thankful I met her and loved her and let her love me.

Writing this made me weep!

Conclusion

I remember one day when Tammy was staring into space and I asked her what was wrong, her response was, "I am sad because I cannot plan anything." I knew that I usually cautioned her about "doing too much," so I sat down in front her and simply said, "You know, you are right. Let's plan anyway. Let's plan a trip and if you are too ill to go, we will just cancel." In that moment, I decided to "get a new bicycle" and look at our situation a little differently. I wanted her to feel like she was able to look forward to her future, even if the future was not very long.

Although Tammy and I have decided to live our lives one day at a time, it is sometimes difficult to do. After our conversation, Tammy immediately began to plan our vacation. The trip Tammy planned was the trip to the beach. The one where I lost my bicycle on the interstate. On that trip, when we arrived at our destination, I bought a new beach cruiser and we did bike all over the beach town. We had a fantastic, relaxing trip! Although I began my story discussing a bicycle, I chose the painting of a bicycle to conclude my story (Figure 6). I did not replace my pink beach cruiser with another pink beach cruiser; I bought a red bicycle as a constant reminder that happiness is found in the ability to be flexible and live in the moment. Over the past year, I have learned how to navigate through endometrial cancer, a devastating diagnosis and prognosis, discrimination, our relationship before and after the diagnosis, self-care, and being forced to consider my life without my wife.

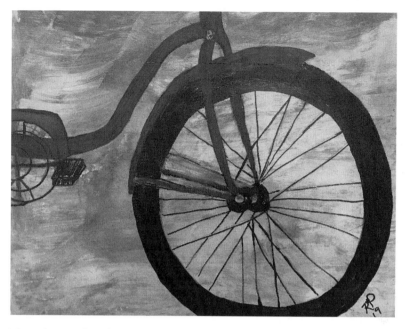

Figure 6. I need a new bicycle.

I am constantly having to relate to my wife in differing ways; my role changes constantly to meet her needs. Although all my conversations have changed and become about cancer, I have learned to cope with all of it and truly live "one day at a time." According to Weingarten and Dulwich Centre Publications (2000), illness narratives take on different forms and one of those forms is a restitution narrative, which is the story of diagnosis, treatment, and prognosis where the storyteller sees the illness as a detour and overcomes the illness. It is the most socially accepted type of illness narrative, because of its positive spin. The second form of illness narrative is a chaos narrative where the narrative is hopeless and jumps around in plotline development. Chaos narratives are difficult to read and hear. The third form is the quest narrative where the storyteller faces her illness head on and deals with the path on which the illness projects. Although our illness narrative could be considered a little bit of all three forms that Weingarten and Dulwich Centre Publications (2000) discusses, I would really like this narrative to be remembered as a story of healing instead of the sadness that a terminal illness has caused my wife and me. I want people to read this and understand that every case is unique, every story is powerful and what Tammy and I have learned about each other is that what we promised on our wedding day was true to us and those words we said have sustained us through all of this. We are a lesbian couple and we are thankful for our right to marry and to take care of each other.

After writing this autoethnography through the act of painting and journaling, I feel it has helped me to have better control of my ability to cope with my everyday life. Individual narratives are important, and it is imperative that therapists honor that uniqueness using alternative methods of expression like painting and journaling or using a metaphor like my bicycle to help them cycle through their own narrative.

Disclouser statement

The author declares that she has no competing interests.

ORCID

Karen Parker ⓘ http://orcid.org/0000-0003-3026-8553

References

Bauer, J. J., & Bonanno, G. A. (2001). Continuity amid discontinuity: Bridging one's past and present in stories of conjugal bereavement. *Narrative Inquiry*, *11*(1), 123–158. https://doi.org/10.1075/ni.11.1.06bau

Chang, H. (2008). *Autoethnography as method*. Left Coast Press.

Creswell, J. W., & Poth, C. N. (2017). *Qualitative inquiry & research design: Choosing among five approaches*. Sage.

Davis, C. G., & Nolen-Hoeksema, S. (2001). Loss and meaning. how do people make sense of loss? *American Behavioral Scientist*, *44*(5), 726–741. https://doi.org/10.1177/0002764201044005003

Ellis, C., & Bochner, A. P. (2000). Autoethnography, personal narrative, reflexivity: Researcher as subject. In N. Denzin & Y. Lincoln (Eds.), *The handbook of qualitative research* (2nd ed., pp. 733–768). Sage.

Fallin-Bennett, K. (2015). Implicit bias against sexual minorities in medicine: Cycles of professional influence and the role of the hidden curriculum. *Academic Medcine.*, *90*(5), 549–552. https://doi.org/10.1097/ACM.0000000000000662

Goff, B. A., Kato, D. D., Schmidt, E. M., Ferry, J. A., Muntz, H. G., Cain, J. M., Tamim, H. K., Figge, D. C., & Greer, B. E. (1994). Uterine papillary serous carcinoma: Patterns of metastatic spread. *Gynecologic Oncology.*, *54*(3), 264–268. https://doi.org/10.1006/gyno.1994.1208

Hall, C. (2014). Bereavement theory: Recent developments in our understanding of grief and bereavement. *Bereavement Care*, *33*(1), 7–12. https://doi.org/10.1080/02682621.2014.902610

Hirsch, O., Löltgen, K., & Becker, A. (2016). Lesbian womens' access to healthcare, experiences with and expectations towards GPs in German primary care. *BMC Family Practice*, *17*(1), 162. https://doi.org/10.1186/s12875-016-0562-4

Human Rights Campaign Foundation. (2019). *Healthcare equality index (2019)*. Human Rights Campaign. https://assets2.hrc.org/files/assets/resources/HEI-2019-FinalReport.pdf

Kübler-Ross, E. (1969). *On death and dying*. The Macmillan Company.

Macy, S. (2011). *Wheels of Change: How Women Rode the Bicycle to Freedom (With a Few Flat Tires Along the Way)*. National Geographic, 2011.

Mizzi, R. (2010). Unraveling researcher subjectivity through multivocality in autoethnography. *Journal of Research Practice*, 6(1), Article M3. http://jrp.icaap.org/index.php/jrp/article/view/201/185

Neville, S., & Henrickson, M. (2006). Perceptions of lesbian, gay and bisexual people of primary healthcare services. *Journal of Advanced Nursing*, 55(4), 407–415. https://doi.org/10.1111/j.1365-2648.2006.03944.x

Sullivan, G. (2008). Painting as research: Create and critique. In G. Knowles & A. Cole (Eds.), *Handbook of arts in qualitative research: Perspectives, methodologies, examples, and issues* (pp. 241–242). Sage Publications..

Weingarten, K. (2000). *The politics of illness narratives: who tells, who listens and who cares in narrative* therapy *and* community work: *A Conference Collection*. Adelaide: Dulwich Centre Publications. In M. White & D. Epston Dulwich Centre Publications (Eds..), *(1990). Narrative means to therapeutic ends* (pp. 13–26). Norton & Company

Williams, R. M. C. (2009). Graphic Historiography: A qualitative research project using Visual Art as a Method of Inquiry and Understanding. AERA Annual Meeting. SIG-Arts and Inquiry in the Visual and Performing Arts in Education. https://doi.org/10.17077/6nvk-fux7

Breast Cancer and Body Image: Feminist Therapy Principles and Interventions

Chiquita Holmes, Alexis Jackson, Joan Looby, Kasia Gallo, and Kendra Blakely

ABSTRACT
A breast cancer diagnosis can lead to life-altering biopsychosocial changes and challenges for breast cancer survivors (BCS). Particularly salient is body image perception and its associated biopsychosocial ramifications. This manuscript examined the impact of breast cancer on women's body image, including women of color and lesbians. The information was contextualized through the application of feminist theory principles. Interventions and implications for breast cancer survivors (BCS) were discussed utilizing feminist theory.

The American Cancer Society identifies breast cancer as the most frequently diagnosed cancer in women. In 2019, approximately 268,600 women will be diagnosed, and 41,760 will die from the disease (American Cancer Society, 2019). Though White women are diagnosed at higher rates, 42% more Black women die of breast cancer compared to White women (Foy et al., 2018). The Centers for Disease Control Prevention's 2016 snapshot of the breast cancer mortality rates among the U.S. female demographic indicates that per 100,000 cases, approximately 27% Black, 20% White, 14% Latina, 12% American Indian/Alaska Native, and 11% Asian/Pacific Islander women in the country die of breast cancer (Center for Disease Control and Prevention, 2016).

A diagnosis of breast cancer has pervasive consequences on a woman's physical and mental health. The breasts signal femininity and are physical emblems of womanhood. However, breast cancer and the associated treatments such as surgery, chemotherapy, and adjunctive hormone therapy, leave a woman physically and psychologically ravaged. The effects of scarring, breast and hair loss, and reduced sexual and reproductive functioning leave her to grapple with issues of body image and previously held ideas of sexuality, femininity, and wholeness as a woman (Boquiren et al., 2013). For this manuscript, data on breast cancer, body image, and their impact on breast cancer survivors (BCS), including the family, are presented and contextualized through the application of feminist theory principles and interventions. Implications for BCS are discussed.

A theoretical framework for understanding breast cancer and body image

Several theories provide a framework for understanding body image difficulties among BCS. The cognitive behavioral model of body image purported by Cash (2011) includes body image evaluation and body image investment. Body image evaluation refers to the degree of satisfaction with one's body and any discrepancies between the real and ideal physical self-image, while body image investment encapsulates the overall physical appearance. Another cognitive behavioral model by White (2002) emphasizes survivor perceptions and experiences of appearance changes, whether those changes are noticeable or not. Changes from breast cancer will result in negative body image depending on the level of body investment and any discrepancy between the real and ideal physical self-image. Fingeret et al. (2013) theoretical framework place body image concerns of BCS on a continuum ranging from mild to extreme. Survivors with more pronounced body image concerns interact less favorably with others and BCS minimize body image difficulties because of shame or embarrassment (Fingeret et al., 2013).

Conceptually, body image includes perceptions, thoughts, feelings, and behaviors related to the body's appearance, functions, and capabilities (Fingeret et al., 2014; Paterson et al., 2016). Negative body image creates lifelong challenges that impact a survivor's recovery. Disease and treatment fallout include appearance alterations, sensory changes, functional impairments, exacerbation of menopausal symptoms, and threats to reproductive capacity (Lewis-Smith et al., 2018). These challenges increase a survivor's psychological vulnerability and result in a plethora of clinical outcomes.

The empirical literature on body image and BCS reveals mixed findings. Researchers have linked a positive body image with increased coping skills, but also reported BCS negative perceptions such as displeasure and insecurity with personal appearance, loss of femininity, physical incompleteness, unwillingness to view their naked form, decreased attractiveness, and discontent with surgical scarring (Pikler & Winterwood, 2003). In other studies, BCS experienced altered views of their bodies and felt less attractive and more disfigured following treatment (Paterson et al., 2016; Van Puymbroeck et al., 2011).

Body image is a very salient concern for younger BCS, and many of the issues with which they struggle involve loss of breasts following surgery (Paterson et al., 2016). The National Cancer Institute estimated that 33% of new breast cancer diagnoses were in women 54 years or younger (Howard-Anderson et al., 2012). Results from a systematic review of 36 body image studies published from 2000–2014 and including 9,343 participants, indicated that younger BCS experienced poorer body image, psychological and physical distress, poorer global health, sexuality and intimacy issues, and poor partnered relationships (Paterson et al., 2016). The researchers concluded that this population's vulnerability to negative treatment effects and aggressive cancers underscores the urgency of developing empirically sound interventions to address body image disturbance.

A related review (Fingeret et al., 2014) included 92 studies published from 2003–2013 on body image difficulties. Findings specific to BCS included increased body image concerns, adverse psychological stress, higher levels of anxiety and depression, lower quality of life, and poorer sexual functioning. Similarly, Rezaei et al. (2016) reviewed 44 published studies from 1993–2016 on factors influencing body image of BCS. The researchers identified bio-psycho-economic, treatment, disease, physical appearance, and sexual functioning factors as impacting BCS psychological functioning and body image.

Researchers also investigated gender socialization and body consciousness on body image disturbance in BCS (Boquiren et al., 2013). They found that BCS who internalized traditional gender roles and attitudes experienced greater body shame and body image disturbance and a poorer quality of life. Similarly, in a study of the quality of life of BCS 4 to 42 months after diagnosis, researchers concluded that younger BCS risk an impaired quality of life for several years after diagnosis (Avis et al., 2005). In another longitudinal study on body image and psychosocial adjustment, Moreira and Canavarro (2010) found that having a mastectomy was associated with shame and lower appearance satisfaction, and initial body image did not affect later body image appearance in BCS.

The literature reviewed substantiated that body image is associated with a variety of adverse outcomes for BCS. It emphasized the need for further research to address negative body image concerns and to design new treatment modalities. Also, methodological issues such as small sample sizes, limited diversity of participants, and variations in assessment tools and research designs (Fingeret et al., 2014; Paterson et al., 2016) impacted the generalizability of the findings.

Biopsychosocial challenges for breast cancer survivors

In addition to body image, BCS struggle with other biopsychosocial issues that affect their diagnosis and treatment. The ramifications place additional stress on BCS and compound an already complex situation. Challenges include financial, physical, sexual, social, and clinical concerns.

Financial instability directly impacts BCS ability to access quality care as well as their survival rates. The loss of economic viability combined with the medical expenses of a breast cancer diagnosis affects not only the BCS but also family members and partners (Rotter et al., 2018). Financial stability is essential for the purposes of extended medical stays, procedures, medications, and co-pays. It is helpful for BCS to have the support of spousal finances and insurance to avoid financial strain. Financial instability is especially taxing on BCS because of the economic hardship, financial distress, and financial burden it causes (Ashing et al., 2018). Insurance concerns and directives present additional obstacles, primarily since levels of coverage differ, health care plans vary, and some BCS cannot afford treatment without insurance (Rotter et al., 2018). Findings from a study on patient recommendations for reducing the financial burden after breast cancer included expansion of insurance and insurance covered items, domestic and financial assistance from diagnosis through treatment, and preserving previous employment (Dean et al., 2019).

BCS also experience a variety of physical changes stemming from breast loss. Resulting concerns include hormone imbalances, hair loss, fluctuations in weight, the development of adjuvant tumors, scarring and disfiguration, nerve damage, and unfavorable skin color changes resulting from chemotherapy and radiation (Boquiren et al., 2013; Lewis-Smith et al., 2018). Research on body image and BCS and the disease and treatment process confirm the above findings (Fingeret et al., 2014; Rezaei et al., 2016). These changes lead to frequent medical crises and uncertainty about surviving.

Struggles with sexuality also plague BCS. In a study of body image and sexual problems in 549 BCS aged 22–50, difficulties related to sexuality, sexual activity, early menopause, body image and physical appearance, poorer mental health, and lack of partners understanding of BCS feelings were reported (Fobair & Spiegel, 2009; Fobair et al., 2006). Related research found that increased preoccupation with body image in younger BCS makes them more amenable to breast reconstruction (Paterson et al., 2016). A relevant study of 90 younger BCS found that those who had mastectomies reported poor sexual functioning, depression, and lower body image than those in the mastectomy reconstruction and control groups (Archangelo et al., 2019).

Nineteen studies on sexual dysfunction published from 2002–2017 were systematically reviewed (Jing et al., 2019) including 2,684 BCS who were administered a brief self-report measure of female sexual function. The researchers reported that women with breast cancer had higher female sexual dysfunction prevalence rates and lower sexual function, and American women with breast cancer had average female sexual dysfunction prevalence and lower average sexual function than Asian women with breast cancer (Jing et al., 2019).

Findings from other studies indicated that BCS in partnered relationships remain sexually active while receiving treatment for their breast cancer; however, many women opt out of sexual encounters, as they are prone to experiencing difficulties with sexual activity, performance, and physical appearance (Fobair et al., 2006; Oberguggenberger et al., 2017). For women in partnered relationships, sexual inadequacy and body unattractiveness inhibited their levels of intimacy and comfort with their sexuality. BCS also struggled with dating, keeping their breast cancer diagnosis a secret, and termination of or change in a partnered relationship (Trachtenberg, 2012).

Social relationships and role strain factors cause additional distress. Protective factors for BCS include family, friends, supportive networks, groups, and professional resources (Campbell-Enns & Woodgate, 2017).

Consequently, if BCS cannot maintain healthy relationships with these communities, it will be difficult for them to adapt to changes brought about by breast cancer. BCS experience alienation from peers who shun them and perceive them as sick because of the fear that accompanies a breast cancer diagnosis (Trachtenberg, 2012). For young BCS, the physical ramifications of treatment create fertility issues (Howard-Anderson et al., 2012). An inability to fulfill maternal tasks has a psychological impact on BCS and reshapes how others view them. Because society associates women with being nurturers who use their breasts for feeding, BCS will feel inadequate if they are unable to execute this role (Boquiren et al., 2013; Inhestern & Bergelt, 2018). For example, a review of 28 articles published from 1990–2010 on quality of life, fertility, and health outcomes in younger breast cancer survivors, indicated that younger BCS experienced more psychosocial and menopausal issues than older BCS. These stressors negatively affected their overall health (Howard-Anderson et al., 2012).

Breast cancer survivors are also at risk for one or more clinical disorders such as post-traumatic stress disorder, depression, anxiety, low self-esteem and self-worth, loneliness, and suicidal ideation (Ashing et al., 2018). BCS most commonly experience depression, which results in a diminished standard of life for one in five BCS (Boing et al., 2019). BCS often fear death, experience a tremendous loss of control, and feel taken prisoner by the illness. Therefore, it is not unusual for BCS to have suicidal thoughts, especially following a mastectomy (Szumacher, 2006). The inability to process the trauma of a breast cancer diagnosis results in emotional dysregulation, frustration, spontaneous emotional outbursts, and mood swings that affect BCS personal, professional, and family relationships (Grecucci et al., 2015).

Women of color and lesbian breast cancer survivors: treatment disparities

It is necessary to understand women of color and lesbian BCS lived experiences. Limited research has indicated that body image concerns are not as critical an issue for women of color BCS because of cultural factors (Ashing-Giwa et al., 2004); however, many of these women have limited economic, physical, social, and psychological resources to aid in their recovery from breast cancer (Ashing et al., 2018). Therefore, they remain underserved and at risk for substandard or no treatment, thereby increasing their mortality rates as confirmed by the Center for Disease Control and Prevention (2016).

Research on women of color and lesbian BCS is limited. Available research outlines a familiar theme, that women of color and lesbian BCS report the poorest results with breast cancer survival rates, body image concerns, and overall psychological distress (Patel-Kerai et al., 2017). Mortality among Black women is more than 40% higher than that of White women, and Black women die from breast cancer due to discontinuation of treatment and late diagnosis

(Richardson et al., 2016). Black and Latina women postpone and ignore mammograms and follow up recommendations for a variety of reasons, thus increasing their risk for more severe types of breast cancer and shorter survival rates (Yedjou et al., 2017). Additionally, cultural mores and crises influence these women's decisions to undergo cancer screenings and treatment (Patel-Kerai et al., 2017).

Latina women BCS are ambivalent regarding screenings and follow-up care, feeling that healing comes from God instead of medical technology, and reported difficulties communicating with their medical provider (Ashing-Giwa et al., 2004). Results of a survey of 6,722 BCS of all racial and ethnic backgrounds indicated that 19% reported communication problems with their providers, and of this 19%, White BCS (16%) had fewer problems than Black (23%) and Latina (33%) BCS. Culture also influences who determines the survivor's healthcare decisions, and many providers seemed to have a standardized format for diagnosis and treatment of breast cancer without considering the women's health literacy and cultural beliefs (King et al., 2008).

> Research on body image across four racial groups (Black, Asian American, Latina and White) revealed that Black and South Asian BCS stated more body image concerns than White women (Patel-Kerai et al., 2017), which is different from results found by (Ashing-Giwa et al., 2004). Further, women from all groups reported challenges adjusting to physical changes from breast cancer, with White women expressing anger and disappointment for getting breast cancer despite their healthy lifestyle. Frequent comments centered on body disgust, decreased self-worth and attractiveness, feeling deformed and inadequate, and a sense of loss.

Ashing-Giwa et al. (2004) conducted a qualitative study of the breast cancer experiences of Black, White, Asian, and Latina BCS. Results indicated that some Black BCS were unwilling to accept their bodies and feared their partner's rejection of their physical appearance; other Black BCS affirmed that breast cancer did not diminish their roles as women, mothers, or wives. Latina BCS worried about weight gain and self-acceptance, while Asian BCS were distressed by their changed bodies. Self-acceptance was more difficult for younger women, and older women viewed their bodies less negatively (Ashing-Giwa et al., 2004).

Boehmer et al. (2013) suggested that resiliency following treatment is higher in lesbian and bisexual survivors, as these survivors use similar coping strategies to navigate both sexual identity discrimination and survivorship (Boehmer et al., 2013). Lesbian BCS are at an increased risk for breast cancer because of less frequent mammogram screenings than cisgender women (Bazzi et al., 2015), extended use of hormones and delay in childbirth (Szumacher, 2006), reduced pregnancy rates (Quinn et al., 2015), and alcohol use, smoking, and obesity (Meads & Moore, 2013). Meads and Moore (2013) reviewed 198 studies on incidence, prevalence rates, and risk studies on breast cancer in lesbians, and bisexual women, and suggested a lack of clarity about higher incidences of breast cancer among lesbians because of the poor methodological quality of the studies. The authors suggested that collecting sexual orientation data from cancer registries or large cohort studies is best (Meads & Moore, 2013). Although it seems that lesbians and bisexual women have an increased prevalence of breast cancer risk factors, it is unclear if they are indeed at an increased risk of breast cancer (Quinn et al., 2015).

Breast cancer contextualized: application and discussion of feminist principles

Cognitive behavioral interventions, guided imagery, psychosexual therapy, cosmetic interventions, massage therapy, yoga, and exercise are cited as interventions for targeting the body image distress of BCS (Fingeret et al., 2014; Lewis-Smith et al., 2018). However, understanding the socio-political context of BCS distress provides additional information about their experiences. Feminist therapy integrates feminist principles into therapeutic interventions and attributes psychological anguish to sociopolitical and cultural contexts instead of women's flaws (Enns, 2012; Evans & Miller, 2015). Two tenets of feminist therapy that provide a framework for contextualizing the experiences of BCS – the personal is political and honoring women's voices Corey (2017) – will be used to illustrate their applicability.

The personal is political

At the core of feminist therapy is the principle that the personal is political (Enns, 2012). It means that women's psychological issues are embedded in the lived values of a patriarchal and gendered society that disempowers and marginalizes them in political, social, cultural, and economic contexts (Enns, 2012; Evans et al., 2010; Evans & Miller, 2015). These contexts are fraught with difficulties surrounding gender roles and expectations, minority status, power differentials, and socialization experiences. Ultimately, the pressures emanating from these experiences manifest themselves into psychological challenges that women continuously confront. Feminist therapy explores how systems of privilege and power block women from achieving their potential and empowers women to make changes in their lives that promote gender equality (Evans et al., 2010; Pusateri & Headley, 2015). The personal is the political manifests in the lives of BCS in several ways.

Women as sex objects

In Western culture, men shape standards for gender role expectations and female attractiveness. Consequently, a woman's appearance is given continuous agency both by men and by women (Boquiren et al., 2013; Corey, 2017; Evans et al., 2010). Women judge themselves and equate their self-worth with unrealistic standards of beauty, while the weight loss, cosmetic and clothing industries continue to profit handsomely from selling "attractiveness" to them. Society has created different rules for men and women around attractiveness, sexuality, and gender roles and expectations. The societal message is that sex and sensuality sell. For BCS who are heavily invested in their appearance, yet do not meet the societal standards of beauty, body image, sexuality, body shame and stigma, and body betrayal are pertinent concerns for them (Trachtenberg, 2012).

Women and imperfect bodies

Societal objectification of the breasts is prevalent. Some BCS have lost both breasts. Because society equates a woman's breasts with her sexuality and womanhood, BCS feel devalued because their bodies are "imperfect" as defined by society (Boquiren et al., 2013). BCS struggle with nursing a child, wearing specific styles of clothing, being afraid to look at the surgical body scars, conflicts about how others perceive their missing breasts, treatment from others, and feeling less than womanly. Further, if the BCS decides against breast reconstructive surgery, they are strongly encouraged to reconsider by loved ones and the medical establishment who regard breast reconstruction as a means of preserving survivors' appearance and restoring normalcy (Rubin & Tanenbaum, 2011; Szumacher, 2006). Younger BCS opt for reconstructive surgery for this reason (Campbell-Enns & Woodgate, 2017). Residual effects of chemotherapy and radiation such as hair loss, skin color changes, and weight fluctuations, also cause significant distress (Lewis-Smith et al., 2018; Przezdziecki et al., 2013). BCS self-esteem and culturally ingrained messages about attractiveness shape their reactions to their altered bodies.

Women as child-bearers

The personal is the political resonates with the deeply imbedded cultural imperative that women are created to bear children (Boquiren et al., 2013). For example, women who have not borne children are frequently questioned about such plans. Even more pronounced are negative societal attitudes about women who choose not to have children. Breast loss, sexual dysfunction, and the inability to bear children represent threats to a woman's femininity and reproductive capability (Boquiren et al., 2013). For BCS of childbearing age, these attitudes impact already existing partnered relationships and prospective future relationships, especially if having children is desired (Avis et al., 2005; Howard-Anderson et al., 2012). Embedded in women's cultural socialization is the notion that fertility and childbearing define their person. Infertility threatens their integrity and sense of self. For BCS, this imperative becomes yet another source of distress and an example of the personal being political.

Breast reconstruction

While breast reconstruction is an elective procedure, many BCS feel pressured by their provider to justify their decision against reconstructive breast surgery (Rubin & Tanenbaum, 2011). Physicians must be careful not to suggest that the woman's physical presentation, specifically her breasts, signal wholeness, physical attractiveness, and femininity. Such action reinforces the dominant culture's perspective and a paternalistic viewpoint. Feminist perspectives call for empowered decision-making and encourage BCS to make their own choices regarding femininity and sexuality (Sulik & Zierkiewicz, 2014). Breast reconstruction is confusing for BCS. Those who decide against it are viewed as de-sexualized; those who chose it, endorse societal norms of attractiveness.

Women's voices are valued and honored

Feminist therapy focuses on honoring the experiences and perspectives of all women, especially those rendered voiceless by marginalization, oppression, and all types of devaluation (Corey, 2017; Enns, 2012). When women are validated, included, speak their truths, make their own choices, and trust their intuition, the gender dialogue shifts to inclusivity and belonging (Evans et al., 2010; Evans & Miller, 2015). The personal becomes political when systemic mechanisms set in place by society continue to give little value to all women's voices. For some BCS, being rendered voiceless is manifested in continued breast cancer treatment disparities, including limited inclusion in cancer trials and research studies, poorer treatment outcomes, and lower breast cancer survival rates.

Limited demographic diversity

Breast cancer studies usually involve White, young, middle-class women who possess the necessary time and participation resources while women from diverse ethnic and socio-economic backgrounds (e.g., older age, women of color, lesbian women, lower socio-economic status, international women) are not frequently included in research protocols and cancer trials (Ashing-Giwa et al., 2004; Meads & Moore, 2013; Rubin & Tanenbaum, 2011; Szumacher, 2006). With data lacking, information on best cancer treatment choices do not include the voices of all women, but just a selected few.

Treatment disparities and survival rates

Black women have higher rates of advanced, aggressive cancer when the cancer is first discovered and higher mortality rates than White women, with a death rate of 42% (DeSantis et al., 2016; Richardson et al., 2016).

Breast cancer is the most common cancer and the leading cause of cancer death among Latina women (Rey-Vargas et al., 2019). Black and Latina women are less likely than White women to be screened for breast cancer, are diagnosed later, and are less likely to receive recommended treatments. Asian/Pacific Islanders and White women are screened for cancer at comparable rates (Chen & Li, 2015). Lesbian women are at a higher risk of developing breast cancer because of reproductive and lifestyle risk factors (Meads & Moore, 2013; Quinn et al., 2015). Further, women 65 and older are less likely to be screened for breast cancer than younger women (Chen & Li, 2015).

Reasons for these health disparities include poverty, communication and language barriers, lack of a primary care provider, lifestyle behavior choices, lack of understanding about healthcare risks, and cultural practices and beliefs (Yedjou et al., 2017). These treatment disparities have impacted the survival rates of women of color and lesbian BCS and represent a serious social justice issue because these women still remain voiceless.

Lack of autonomy and participation in treatment

Shared decision-making represents the gold standard of patient care, where BCS and their medical providers are intimately involved in treatment protocols and outcomes (Rubin & Tanenbaum, 2011; Szumacher, 2006). For some BCS, such participation presents a variety of challenges. Roadblocks such as social class and cultural difficulties, sexual orientation, communication and language challenges, misunderstanding about healthcare risks and cultural practices, provider insensitivity, systemic insensitivity, negative contact with providers, and paternalistic providers, compromise quality care (Ashing-Giwa et al., 2004; Sulik & Zierkiewicz, 2014; Szumacher, 2006). These factors reinforce BCS invisibility in marginalized populations.

Treatment disparities exist among specific communities of BCS and encompass layers of social, psychological, cultural/ethnic, and economic variables. Culturally appropriate, relevant health care must be a right for all BCS and must address the biopsychosocial and cultural barriers outlined that prevent these women from accessing proper care. Listening to and honoring the voices of BCS are powerful treatment tools for accessing their journeys, planning treatment needs, and increasing their survival rates.

Clinical interventions for breast cancer survivors utilizing feminist therapy principles

Gender role analysis

Gender role analysis invites women to explore gender socialization practices on their identities, personhood, and power, including direct and indirect messages focused on "appropriate" gender behaviors, values, and expectations (Corey, 2017; Enns, 2012; Evans & Miller, 2015). Therapists encourage BCS to identify positive and negative messages they receive about beauty, body image, sexuality, and gender role expectations from family, society, and the environment. The information will inform BCS experiences with breast cancer by illustrating how socialization practices have influenced their breast cancer survivorship. Therapists consider asking questions such as: "How did you learn about gender?" "What did you learn about gender?" "In what ways does this information help you to understand your breast cancer experiences?" This dialogue will open up more in-depth exploration to include additional queries on beauty and attractiveness, body image, and sexuality.

Therapists and BCS jointly explore the meanings of health and illness and definitions of attractiveness from a cultural and individual perspective to help BCS distinguish between their own beliefs and those of society (Trachtenberg, 2012). Exploring BCS lived experiences of these meanings gives voice to their truths conceptualized through the lenses of their journey instead of society's narrative.

Reinforcing existing power imbalances and gender role expectations lead to faulty thinking. To address this, therapists and BCS collaborate to identify situations that challenged the BCS core beliefs about gender and role intersectionality. Therapists can teach BCS through empowerment skills, how to change those situations and make new choices. Most importantly, therapists can help BCS understand that even though their experiences were influenced by a society where gender role expectations are ingrained and sometimes difficult to change, BCS have the power to rewrite their individual stories. They are not stuck and can redefine themselves by creating an "after breast cancer" identity that currently defines them.

Gender role intervention

Gender role intervention emphasizes ways that societal gender expectations exacerbate and reinforce distress (Corey, 2017; Enns, 2012; Evans & Miller, 2015). For BCS, distress results from a variety of factors, including the inability to bear children, not conforming to cultural standards of beauty or role strain caused by the debilitating effects of breast cancer (Campbell-Enns & Woodgate, 2017; Howard-Anderson et al., 2012). BCS hear these messages directly, indirectly, and continuously that stepping out of their prescribed roles is not acceptable.

BCS blame themselves for their difficulties instead of looking at external factors. Therapists assist BCS in understanding that their psychological pain is environmentally constructed. When therapists couch distress as caused externally by unjust systems instead of internal flaws, BCS feel less self-blame for their intrapsychic difficulties. Therapists also explain to BCS that they believed these messages because of powerlessness, lack of resources, lack of a voice, societal dictates, or conditioning. By contextualizing BCS experiences in this manner, therapists encourage them to create new messages that are more positive, realistic, empowering, and honest.

Power analysis

Power analysis allows BCS to understand how gendered power differentials limit women's well-being, self-development, choices, and potential (Enns, 2012; Pusateri & Headley, 2015). These power imbalances manifest in a variety of ways including body image concerns, stereotypical gender roles, discrimination, minimal resources, demographic disparities (e.g., race, sexual minority status, age, class, socio-economic status, culture), whether or not to have reconstructive surgery, making treatment decisions, and selecting a provider (Campbell-Enns & Woodgate, 2017; Fingeret et al., 2014; Howard-Anderson et al., 2012; Rubin & Tanenbaum, 2011; Szumacher, 2006). Therapists support the BCS in identifying power they already have but are not aware, and dialogue about how that power can be used to challenge oppressive systems that impact BCS. For example, conversations about decision-making, goal setting, identifying their existing power despite the diagnosis, empowering and supporting their choices to change insensitive providers, refusing reconstructive surgery, and refusing to wear a wig, are compelling. Helping BCS to celebrate their lived experiences and accept their identities as survivors within the context of their own instead of society's expectations, are ways to regain power and create change.

Consciousness raising

Consciousness raising, a principle of feminist therapy, provides a venue for women to create awareness of their experiences with gender-based discrimination, oppression, devaluation, and marginalization (Enns, 2012; Evans & Miller, 2015). It allows women to distinguish between socially dictated and health behavioral choices and to make choices consistent with their needs and desires (Evans et al., 2010; Evans & Miller, 2015). Consciousness raising allows women to share their truths. Consciousness raising groups provide support, camaraderie, commonality of experiences, and linkages to mechanisms for changing oppressive social structures (Corey, 2017; Enns, 2012). Therapists discuss with BCS the benefits of joining such a group. Particularly for BCS who feel voiceless, these groups allow universality of experiences with other survivors, automatic network support, decreased isolation, and opportunities for catharsis (Corey, 2017; Enns, 2012). In addition to consciousness raising groups, therapists refer BCS to specialized groups and organizations that provide support for cancer survivors or to long-term therapy. Diverse women's voices at the center of therapy offer a variety of perspectives, experiences, and truths.

Reframing and relabeling

Feminist therapists view clinical diagnosis as an artifact of patriarchy and conceptualize mental health concerns as the result of intrapsychic issues resulting from socially and culturally imposed systems (Enns, 2012; Evans & Miller, 2015). Therapists reframe psychological distress as a reaction to coping in a stressful, socio-political, and hostile environment, and a conditioned response to oppressive factors (Enns, 2012). Reframing and relabeling moves from blaming the woman to examining social systems and elements in the environment that are responsible (Enns, 2012; Evans & Miller, 2015). For example, if a survivor is experiencing depression and negative body image concerns from breast cancer surgery, the therapist reframes the problem by saying that her angst is a result of society's focus on ideal standards of beauty defined by men, and not an intrapsychic deficiency. Similarly, relabeling retitles the behavior – the BCS repeats to herself that she is courageous for having undergone breast cancer surgery, or she is strong for choosing not to have reconstructive breast surgery. Therapists reinforce and relabel behaviors so that BCS do not internalize unfair societal imperatives.

Commitment to social change

Feminist therapists aim for social change (Corey, 2017; Enns, 2012; Evans & Miller, 2015). Therapists discuss with BCS how their identities (race, gender, sexual orientation, religion) have caused oppressive suffering intersecting with their experiences with breast cancer. As members of a marginalized group, BCS join with others to address similar concerns. Advocacy is critical to feminist therapy because personal freedom cannot occur without social change (Enns, 2012; Evans & Miller, 2015). Therapists help BCS to identify their individual advocacy interests and initiatives and use their extensive knowledge to direct BCS to a variety of resources. Some advocacy platforms include volunteering, lobbying activities, community breast cancer education, conference presentations on surviving breast cancer, and conducting and presenting breast cancer research.

Empowerment through photovoice

Photovoice empowers BCS to shape their personal breast cancer narrative through the use of photographs (Liebenberg, 2018; Wang & Burris, 1994). Photovoice is done through recording images that depict common problems, evaluating dialogue around the issues, and using the information to implement change. Photovoice is used to explore many facets of breast cancer and body image. For example, the photographs capture snapshots that are meaningful to survivors, such as their hair growing back in stages, chemotherapy treatments, and pictures of their scars. Discussing the pictures as part of therapy enhances BCS's ability to express their needs and emotions and gives voice to their voice. This technique allows therapists to contextualize BCS feelings better and strengthen the therapeutic support by negotiating the challenges of breast cancer and body image (Sloan et al., 2018). Photovoice promotes the precepts of feminist theory as it provides a vehicle to recognize, analyze, and challenge oppressive systems that influence breast cancer treatment and body image (Mayfield-Johnson et al., 2014).

Self-advocacy and treatment navigation

Individualized psychoeducation and negotiating the healthcare system are paramount when seeking to empower and inform BCS (Freeman & Rodriguez, 2011). Therapists are encouraged to coordinate care with the oncologist and other medical providers. The process will support the continuity of care received by BCS, allow therapists to assist BCS in understanding the role of the medical team, empower survivors to self-advocate any treatment concerns, and reframe the pathology-oriented processes of the medical model of care (Szumacher, 2006). Treatment navigation is used by multidisciplinary medical teams to guide patient care, eliminate barriers to resources, and encourage expedient diagnosis and treatment through a public intervention service. Treatment navigation with the therapist helps BCS avoid barriers related to access, quality of care, communication, financial limitations, and mistrust of the medical community (Freeman & Rodriguez, 2011). It is important that therapists understand strategies that support successful treatment navigation and convey them to BCS. For example, therapists can teach BCS assertiveness skills that facilitate self-guided healthcare and personal advocacy.

Helping medical providers understand the sociopolitical contexts of breast cancer

The multidisciplinary treatment team approach brings together varying disciplines to provide comprehensive medical care to BCS. The treatment team approach demonstrates an orientation similar to that of feminist theory. Both encourage a multidisciplinary strength-focused approach, value diverse perspectives, and are focused on creating egalitarian relationships (Shao et al., 2019). Therapists can help the team to identify the parallel goals that exist between feminist theory and the treatment team model of patient care. Understanding these similarities can help the team more readily identify and contextualize existing sociopolitical aspects of treatment in both a broad and specific patient context. In a broad context, therapists support the treatment team in understanding how social constructs, including race and gender, dictate which disorders are researched, what treatment is available, and where access to treatment is provided (Rogers & Kelly, 2011). In a specific context, therapists outline the survivor's individualized needs with respect to the distribution of power in the patient-physician relationship, traditional perceptions of gender roles, as well as socio-economic status and other disenfranchising systems that impact the treatment process (Sulik & Zierkiewicz, 2014).

Further, when participating with the treatment team, therapists can suggest the implementation of several strategies that promote increased survivorship. Kline et al. (2018) outlined recommendations to support BCS that include integrative psychological care, accessible and cost-effective primary and palliative services, and the development and education of staff that promote person-centered coordinated care. Incorporating feminist theory into treatment planning and decision-making models for BCS gives therapists the opportunity to share resources and education on a variety of issues while improving the overall quality of care BCS receive. Therapists can provide information regarding constructs of power and patient choice. In this forum, therapists can also challenge normative ideas about family, gender, and other sociopolitical concerns that arise (Szumacher, 2006).

Implications for practice

BCS experience life-altering body image and biopsychosocial changes that come with a diagnosis of breast cancer. There are several implications for practitioners beyond the interventions described previously. First, improved continuity of care and integrative treatment planning that addresses not only the medical but also the body image, biopsychosocial, and cultural needs of BCS must become the standard of care. If not, then adequate treatment will continue to be reserved for a select few survivors. Additionally, cultural competency training to ensure appropriate clinical care and understanding of factors responsible for the high mortality rates among underrepresented BCS is essential. Finally, practitioners are called to lend their voices to collaborative grassroots efforts, community campaigns, public health initiatives, and educational partnerships that address the needs of marginalized BCS. This will help to improve BCS quality of life and survival rates.

Limitations and future research

There are several limitations to this manuscript. First, the information is not generalizable to all breast cancer survivors (e.g., men, older women, ethnically and sexually diverse women, women of lower SES). Another major limitation is that much of the extant literature on BCS, including data in this manuscript, focused on young Caucasian BCS and lacks a balanced, diverse perspective (Ashing-Giwa et al., 2004; Fingeret et al., 2013; Paterson et al., 2016); therefore, its applicability to women of diverse demographics is limited. Research continues to outline the disparities in breast cancer and risk factor rates, especially among racial and ethnic minority women. Increased research is necessary to understand the causes of the disparities and how to reduce them so that all women have access to culturally appropriate and effective breast cancer treatment. Additionally, BCS lived experiences can be very dissimilar across identities, and body image may not be an integral concern as highlighted. Finally, this was not an empirical study; therefore, research focusing on BCS utilizing empirically sound methodology, addressing treatment and body image disparities, and focusing on culturally relevant treatment protocols and interventions for BCS is vital. Research through the feminist lens honoring the experiences and voices of a broad spectrum of BCS provides practitioners with a better understanding of the challenges and additional factors to consider for treatment and survivorship.

Conclusion

A breast cancer diagnosis carries medical and biopsychosocial challenges that encompass more than body image concerns. Despite existing research, specific populations of BCS remain underserved, as evidenced by their increased mortality rates and limited inclusion in research. Gaps in research, funding, and educational initiatives still exist. Thus, practitioners who work with BCS are responsible for providing competent, quality, culturally sensitive clinical and therapeutic care, while exploring a variety of initiatives designed to increase BCS life satisfaction and survival rates. Addressing these gaps is not only a feminist therapy imperative but also a social justice responsibility.

References

American Cancer Society. (2019). *Cancer facts & figures 2019*. https://www.cancer.org/content/dam/cancer-org/research/cancer-facts-and-statistics/annual-cancer-facts-and-figures/2019/cancer-facts-and-figures-2019.pdf

Archangelo, S., Sabino, N., Veiga, D., Garcia, E., & Ferreira, L. (2019). Sexuality, depression, and body image after breast reconstruction. *Clinics (Sao Paulo, Brazil), 74*, 883–888. https://doi.org/10.6061/clinics/2019/e883

Ashing, K. T., George, M., & Jones, V. (2018). Health-related quality of life and care satisfaction outcomes: Informing psychosocial oncology care among Latina and African-American young breast cancer survivors. *Psycho-Oncology, 27*(4), 1213–1220. https://doi.org/10.1002/pon.4650

Ashing-Giwa, K. T., Padilla, G., Tejero, J., Kraemer, J., Wright, K., Coscarelli, A., Clayton, S., Williams, I., & Hills, D. (2004). Understanding the breast cancer experience of women: A qualitative study of African American, Asian American, Latina, and White cancer survivors. *Psycho-Oncology, 13*(6), 408–428. https://doi.org/10.1002/pon.750

Avis, N., Crawford, S., & Manuel, J. (2005). Quality of life among younger women with breast cancer. *Journal of Clinical Oncology, 23*(5), 3322–3330. https://doi.org/10.1200/JCO.2005.05.130

Bazzi, A. R., Whorms, D. S., King, D. S., & Potter, J. (2015). Adherence to mammography screening guidelines among transgender persons and sexual minority women. *American Journal of Public Health, 105*(11), 2356–2358. https://doi.org/10.2105/AJPH.2015.302851

Boehmer, U., Glickman, M., Winter, M., & Clark, M. A. (2013). Lesbian and bisexual women's adjustment after a breast cancer diagnosis. *Journal of the American Psychiatric Nurses Association, 19*(5), 280–292. https://doi.org/10.1177/1078390313504587

Boing, L., Pereira, G. S., Araújo, C., Sperandio, F. F., Loch, M., Bergmann, A., & Guimarães, A. (2019). Factors associated with depression symptoms in women after breast cancer. *Revista De Saúde Pública, 53*, 1–12. https://doi.org/10.11606/s1518-8787.2019053000786

Boquiren, V. M., Esplen, M. J., Wong, J., Toner, B., & Warner, E. (2013). Exploring the influence of gender-role socialization and objectified body consciousness on body image disturbance in breast cancer survivors. *Psycho-Oncology, 22*(10), 2177–2185. https://doi.org/10.1002/pon.3271

Campbell-Enns, H. J., & Woodgate, R. L. (2017). The psychosocial experiences of women with breast cancer across the lifespan: A systematic review. *Psycho-Oncology, 26*(11), 1711–1721. https://doi.org/10.1002/pon.4281

Cash, T. F. (2011). Cognitive-behavioral perspectives on body image. In *Body image: A handbook of science, practice, and prevention* (2nd ed., pp. 39–47). Guilford Press.

Center for Disease Control and Prevention. (2016). *Female rate of cancer deaths by race/ethnicity*. https://gis.cdc.gov/Cancer/USCS/DataViz.html

Chen, L., & Li, C. (2015). Racial disparities in breast cancer diagnosis and treatment by hormone receptor and HER2 status. *Cancer Epidemiology and Prevention Biomarkers, 24*(11), 1666–1672. https://dio.org/10.1158/1055-9965.EPI-15-0293

Corey, G. (2017). Feminist therapy. In *Theory and practice of counseling and psychotherapy* (9th ed., pp. 343–354). Cengage Learning.

Dean, L. T., Moss, S. L., Rollinson, S. I., Jaramillo, L. F., Paxton, R. J., & Owczarzak, J. T. (2019). Patient recommendations for reducing long-lasting economic burden after breast cancer. *Cancer, 125*(11), 1929–1940. https://doi.org/10.1002/cncr.32012

DeSantis, C., Fedewa, S., Sauer, A., Kramer, J., Smith, R., & Jemal, A. (2016). Breast cancer statistics, 2015: Convergence of incidence rates between Black and White women. *CA: A Cancer Journal for Clinicians, 66*(1), 31–42. https://doi.org/10.3322/caac.21320

Enns, C. (2012). Feminist approaches to counseling. InE. Altmaier & J. Hansen (Eds.), *The Oxford handbook of counseling psychology* (pp. 434–459). Oxford University Press.

Evans, K., & Miller, M. (2015). Feminist therapy. In I. Marini & M. Stebnicki (Eds.), *The professional counselor's desk reference* (2nd ed., pp. 247–251). Springer Publishing.

Evans, K., Kincade, E., & Seem, S. (2010). *Introduction to feminist therapy: Strategies for social and individual change*. Sage Publishing.

Fingeret, M. C., Nipomnick, S. W., Crosby, M. A., & Reece, G. P. (2013). Developing a theoretical framework to illustrate associations among patient satisfaction, body image, and quality of life for women undergoing breast reconstruction. *Cancer Treatment Reviews, 39*(6), 673–681. https://doi.org/http://doi:10.1016/j.ctrv.2012.12.010

Fingeret, M. C., Teo, I., & Epner, D. E. (2014). Managing body image difficulties of adult cancer patients: Lessons from available research. *Cancer, 120*(5), 633–641. https://doi.org/10.1002/cncr.28469

Fobair, P., & Spiegel, D. (2009). Concerns about sexuality after breast cancer. *Cancer Journal, 15*(1), 19–26. https://doi.org/10.1097/PPO.0b013e31819587bb

Fobair, P., Stewart, S. L., Chang, S., D'Onofrio, C., Banks, P. J., & Bloom, J. R. (2006). Body image and sexual problems in young women with breast cancer. *Psycho-Oncology, 15*(7), 579–594. https://doi.org/10.1002/pon.991

Foy, K., Fisher, J., Lustberg, M., Gray, D., DeGraffinreid, C., & Paskett, E. (2018). Disparities in breast cancer tumor characteristics, treatment, time to treatment, and survival probability among African American and White women. *NPJ Breast Cancer, 4*(1), 1–6. https://doi.org/10.1038/s41523-018-0059-5

Freeman, H., & Rodriguez, R. (2011). History and principles of patient navigation. *Cancer, 117*(15), 3537–3540. https://doi.org/10.1002/cncr.26262

Grecucci, A., Pappaianni, E., Siugzdaite, R., Theuninck, A., Frederick, J., & Job, R. (2015). Mindful emotion regulation: Exploring the neurocognitive mechanisms behind mindfulness. *BioMed-Research International, 2015*, 1–9. https://doi.org/10.1155/2015/670724

Howard-Anderson, J., Ganz, P. A., Bower, J. E., & Stanton, A. L. (2012). Quality of life, fertility concerns, and behavioral health outcomes in younger breast cancer survivors: A systematic review. *Journal of the National Cancer Institute, 104*(5), 386–405. https://doi.org/10.1093/jnci/djr541

Inhestern, L., & Bergelt, C. (2018). When a mother has cancer: Strains and resources of affected families from the mother's and father's perspective - A qualitative study. *BMC Women's Health, 18*(1), 1–11. https://doi.org/10.1186/s12905-018-0562-8

Jing, L., Zhang, C., Li, W., Jin, F., & Wang, A. (2019). Incidence and severity of sexual dysfunction among women with breast cancer: A meta-analysis based on female sexual function index. *Supportive Care in Cancer, 27*(4), 1171–1180. https://doi.org/10.1007/s00520-019-04667-7

King, R. K., Alexander, R. G., Tan-Gregory, A., Donahue, E. J., Kimbrough-Sugick, & Betancourt, J. R. (2008). A plan for action: Key perspectives from the racial/ethnic disparities strategy forum. *Milbank Quarterly, 86*(2), 241–272. https://doi.org/10.1111/j.1468-0009.2008.00521.x

Kline, R. M., Arora, N. K., Bradley, C. J., Brauer, E. R., Graves, D. L., Lunsford, N. B., McCabe, M., Nasso, S., Nekhlyudov, L., Rowland, J., Schear, R., & Ganz, P. (2018). Long-term survivorship care after cancer treatment-summary of a 2017 national cancer policy forum workshop. *Journal of the National Cancer Institute, 110*(12), 1300–1310. https://doi.org/10.1093/jnci/djy176

Lewis-Smith, H., Diedrichs, P. C., & Harcourt, D. (2018). A pilot study of a body image intervention for breast cancer survivors. *Body Image, 27*, 21–31. https://doi.org/10.1016/j.bodyim.2018.08.006

Liebenberg, L. (2018). Thinking critically about photovoice: Achieving empowerment and social change. *International Journal of Qualitative Methods, 17*(1), 1–9. https://doi.org/10.1177/1609406918757631

Mayfield-Johnson, S., Rachal, J. R., & Butler, J., III. (2014). "When we learn better, we do better:" Describing changes in empowerment through photovoice among community health advisors in a breast and cervical cancer health promotion program in Mississippi and Alabama. *Adult Education Quarterly, 64*(2), 91–109. https://doi.org/10.1177/0741713614521862

Meads, C., & Moore, D. (2013). Breast cancer in lesbians and bisexual women: Systematic review of incidence, prevalence, and risk studies. *BMC Public Health, 13*(1), 1–11. https://doi.org/10.1186/1471-2458-13-1127

Moreira, H., & Canavarro, M. C. (2010). A longitudinal study about body image and psychosocial adjustment of breast cancer patients during the course of the disease. *European Journal of Oncology Nursing, 14*(4), 263–270. https://doi.org/10.1016/j.ejon.2010.04.001

Obergguggenberger, A., Martini, C., Huber, N., Fallow, L., Hubalek, M., Daniaux, M., Meraner, V., Holzner, B., Sztankay, M., Gamper, E., & Meraner, V. (2017). Self-reported sexual health: Breast cancer survivors compared to women from the general population – An observational study. *BMC Cancer, 17*(1), 1–9. https://doi.org/10.1186/s12885-017-3580-2

Patel-Kerai, G., Harcourt, D., Rumsey, N., Naqvi, H., & White, P. (2017). The psychosocial experiences of breast cancer amongst Black, South Asian and White survivors: Do differences exist between ethnic groups? *Psycho-Oncology, 26*(4), 515–522. https://doi.org/10.1002/pon.4187

Paterson, C. L., Lengacher, C. A., Donovan, K. A., Kip, K. E., & Tofthagen, C. S. (2016). Body image in younger breast cancer survivors: A systematic review. *Cancer Nursing, 39*(E39–), E58. https://doi.org/10.1186/s12885-017-3580-2

Pikler, V., & Winterwood, C. (2003). Racial and body image differences in coping for women diagnosed with breast cancer. *Health Psychology., 22*(6), 632–637. https://doi.org/10.1037/0278-6133.22.6.632

Przezdziecki, A., Sherman, K. A., Baillie, A., Taylor, A., Foley, E., & Stalgis-Balinski, K. (2013). My changed body: Breast cancer, body image, distress, and self-compassion. *Psycho-Oncology, 22*(8), 1872–1879. https://doi.org/10.1002/pon.3230

Pusateri, C., & Headley, C. (2015). Feminist therapy. In E. Neukrug (Ed.), *The sage encyclopedia of theory in counseling and psychotherapy* (pp. 414–419). Sage Publications.

Quinn, G. P., Sanchez, J. A., Sutton, S. K., Vadaparampil, S. T., Nguyen, G. T., Green, B. L., Kanetsky, P. A., & Schabath, M. B. (2015). Cancer and lesbian, gay, bisexual, transgender/transsexual,and queer/questioning (LGBTQ) populations. *CA: A Cancer Journal for Clinicians, 65*(5), 384–400. https://doi.org/10.3322/caac.21288

Rey-Vargas, L., Sanabria-Salas, C., Fejerman, L., & Serrano-Gómez, S. (2019). Risk factors for triple-negative breast cancer among Latina women. *Cancer Epidemiology and Prevention Biomarkers, 28*(11), 1771–1783. https://doi.org/10.1158/1055-9965.EPI-19-0035

Rezaei, M., Elyasi, F., Janbabai, G., Moosazadeh, M., & Hamzehgardeshi, Z. (2016). Factors influencing body image in women with breast cancer: A comprehensive literature review. *Iranian Red Crescent Medical Journal, 18*(10), 1–28. https://doi.org/10.5812/ircmj.39465

Richardson, L., Henley, J., Miller, J., Massetti, G., & Thomas, C. (2016). Patterns and trends in Black-White differences in breast cancer incidence and mortality - United States, 1999 – 2013. *MMWR, 65*(40), 1093–1098. https://doi.org/10.15585/mmwr.mm6540a1

Rogers, J., & Kelly, U. A. (2011). Feminist intersectionality: Bringing social justice to health disparities research. *Nursing Ethics, 18*(3), 397–407. https://doi.org/10.1177/0969733011398094

Rotter, J., Spencer, J. C., & Wheeler, S. B. (2018). Financial toxicity in advanced and metastatic cancer: Overburdened and underprepared. *Journal of Oncology Practice, 15*(4), 300–307. https://doi.org/10.1200/JOP.18.00518

Rubin, L. R., & Tanenbaum, M. (2011). "Does that make me a woman?": Breast cancer, mastectomy, and breast reconstruction decisions among sexual minority women. *Psychology of Women Quarterly, 35*(3), 401–414. https://doi.org/10.1177/0361684310395606

Shao, J., Rodrigues, M., Corter, A. L., & Baxter, N. N. (2019). Multidisciplinary care of breast cancer patients: A scoping review of multidisciplinary styles, processes, and outcomes. *Current Oncology, 26*(3), 385–397. https://doi.org/10.3747/co.26.4713

Sloan, S., Teti, M., & Benson, J. (2018). Redefining body image after breast cancer: A photovoice study. *Innovation in Aging, 2*(suppl_1), 275–276. https://doi.org/10.1093/geroni/igy023.1019

Sulik, G., & Zierkiewicz, E. (2014). Gender, power, and feminisms in breast cancer advocacy: Lessons from the United States and Poland. *Journal of Gender and Power, 1*(1), 111–145.

Szumacher, E. (2006). The feminist approach in the decision-making process for treatment of women with breast cancer. *Annals-Academy of Medicine Singapore, 35*(9), 655–661.

Trachtenberg, L. (2012). *Identity reformulation among young women with breast cancer* [Doctoral dissertation]. https://tspace.library.utoronto.ca/bitstream/1807/33678/3/Trachtenberg_Lianne_201211_MA_thesis.pdf

Van Puymbroeck, M., Schmid, A., Shinew, K. J., & Hsieh, P. C. (2011). Influence of hatha yoga on physical activity constraints, physical fitness, and body image of breast cancer survivors: A pilot study. *International Journal of Yoga Therapy, 21*(1), 49–60. https://doi.org/10.17761/ijyt.21.1.n852143rv21x188u

Wang, C., & Burris, M. A. (1994). Empowerment through photo novella: Portraits of participation. *Health Education Quarterly, 21*(2), 171–186. https://doi.org/10.1177/109019819402100204

White, C. A. (2002). Body images in oncology. In C. Baker & E. Wertheim (Eds.), *Body image: A handbook of theory, research, and clinical practice* (pp. 379–386). The Guilford Press. https://10.1080/1064026039021873

Yedjou, C., Tchounwou, B., Payton, M., Miele, L., Fonseca, D., Lowe, L., & Alo, R. (2017). Assessing the racial and ethnic disparities in breast cancer mortality in the United States. *International Journal of Environmental Research and Public Health, 14*(5), 486–498. https://doi.org/10.3390/ijerph14050486

Therapeutic Interventions with Families of Breast Cancer Survivors

Alexis Jackson, Chiquita Holmes, Joan Looby, and Kendra Blakely

ABSTRACT
A breast cancer diagnosis presents daunting challenges and disruptions to everyday life for family members and caregivers of breast cancer survivors (BCS). Particularly critical to families are their coping mechanisms, patterns of resiliency, and resource availability to navigate such a transformational experience. Family therapy and family therapists can introduce vulnerable families to a variety of clinical interventions that can be helpful in reducing the distress engendered by a breast cancer diagnosis. This manuscript describes clinical dynamics, considerations, and interventions that can be utilized with families of breast cancer survivors. Implications for practice, limitations, and ideas for future research are discussed.

A breast cancer diagnosis presents formidable challenges to the families of Breast Cancer Survivors (BCS). The diagnosis impacts each family differently depending on the stage and phase of the illness and treatment, the prognosis for survival, challenges accessing treatment, cultural beliefs, economic resources (e.g., insurance and treatment availability and affordability, BCS ability to work after diagnosis), spiritual beliefs, and the family emotional climate and structure (Ng et al., 2017; Rolland et al., 1999; Snyder & Pearse, 2010; Vrontaras, 2018). Common family adaptations focus on role changes, caregiver stressors, financial difficulties, BCS adhering to treatment protocols, communicating with and navigating a variety of medical systems, and developing coping strategies for real and imagined losses (Ruddy & McDaniel, 2013; Snyder & Pearse, 2010; Stenberg et al., 2010; Vrontaras, 2018). Family therapists provide interventions that support the family as they navigate these challenges. This manuscript is Part II of an earlier manuscript entitled, "Breast Cancer and Body Image: Feminist Therapy Principles and Interventions." While the first manuscript was theoretically focused, this manuscript provides useful clinical interventions for BCS and their families, framed through feminist therapy principles.

The therapeutic assistance provided to family members will depend on the family's needs and treatment stage; therefore, therapeutic flexibility is necessary. In the early stages of treatment, strategies focused on accepting the diagnosis, information gathering, renegotiation of roles and responsibilities, restoring family equilibrium, and emotional stabilization are necessary (Sherman & Simonton, 1999). Similarly, in later stages of treatment or if the BCS is terminal, strategies focused on grief and loss, treatment decisions, quality of life, living wills and advanced directives, life reviews and confronting mortality, become more relevant (Rolland et al., 1999; Sherman & Simonton, 1999).

Feminist therapy is efficacious from the initial stage of treatment through the terminal stage, as the foundational tenets build upon an egalitarian therapeutic relationship that positions the family as the expert. The family is empowered through strength-based strategies to define treatment needs from their unique perspectives, to challenge gender-role expectations, and to addresses implications of the breast cancer diagnosis from political, social, and cultural domains.

For this manuscript, interventions focused on assessing the family climate, providing support and educational resources, and communication skills and strategies are presented first. These are followed by strategies addressing structural and organizational challenges and caregiver role strain, existential concerns, grieving losses, and family self-care. Then, expressive arts and mind-body applications are presented. Finally, implications for practice, limitations, and suggestions for future research are offered.

Joining and assessing the family climate

The family therapist's qualities and skills in developing a positive therapeutic relationship are integral to treatment. This section examines useful clinical competencies for joining and assessing the family climate.

The family's cooperation and support will enhance treatment outcomes for the BCS, as family systems resources and support are key to breast cancer survivorship (Northouse et al., 2010; Radina & Armer, 2001; Snyder & Pearse, 2010). Additionally, if the family has encountered difficulties navigating and negotiating existing treatment systems for the BCS, the family therapist must be seen as an ally. If not, the family will be reluctant to access therapy or may not return for a second visit. Therefore, the family therapist must communicate competencies such as empathic understanding, relationship building skills, respect, resourcefulness, and comfort with issues of grief and loss (Sherman & Simonton, 1999). Further, the family may have variable patterns of access and disengagement from therapy. Because utilization rests on specific needs at different stages of breast cancer, the family therapist draws from feminist therapy and establishes an egalitarian therapeutic relationship, with an open-door policy that respects the family's autonomy and decision-making skills and puts therapeutic control in the family's hands (Corey, 2017; Ruddy & McDaniel, 2013).

Assessing the family climate and current levels of functioning are critical intervention tasks for the family therapist. Assessment includes information about the stage, type and phase of the breast cancer, current treatment, current BCS functioning (e.g., social, physical, psychological) and any co-occurring medical conditions (Sherman & Simonton, 1999). Additional information on available resources (e.g., social, psychological, logistical, educational), family coping, family functioning styles, and family structure (disengaged, enmeshed or cohesive) are integral to guiding treatment (Diallo et al., 2019; Radina & Armer, 2001; Rolland et al., 1999; Snyder & Pearse, 2010). The family therapist uses this data to ascertain where to join the family, what their needs are, how to address their needs at different phases of treatment, and to set reasonable therapeutic goals. By doing so, the family therapist uses feminist principles that value the perspectives and experiences of the BCS and family members.

An important goal in the early phase of therapy is for the family members to articulate their emotional journey with the diagnosis. The family therapist is uniquely trained to facilitate this narrative. According to Ruddy and McDaniel (2013), stories cover the breast cancer onset and symptoms, feelings about hearing the diagnosis, the family's response to the diagnosis, causes of the cancer, and accessing successful treatment. The narrative also includes the impact of the cancer on the family, cultural interpretations of the cancer, attitudes about healing and death, spiritual beliefs, and the BCS current condition (Goldenberg et al., 2017; Rolland et al., 1999; Ruddy & McDaniel, 2013).

Consistent with feminist therapy principles, the family therapist encourages family members to share and value diverse perspectives, including feelings and fears about the BCS treatment outcomes (Corey, 2017; Rolland et al., 1999; Sherman & Simonton, 1999). Through these conversations, family members voice their feelings, determine what they can and cannot control, and work to restore family stability and equilibrium (Ruddy & McDaniel, 2013). Such conversations help the family externalize the cancer and coalesce toward a common goal of supporting the BCS through the challenges of treatment.

Because family members of BCS are unprepared for the diagnosis, they may struggle with emotions such as guilt, depression, sorrow, anxiety, denial, grief, anger, and resentment of the family member for getting cancer (Mitschke, 2008; Sherman & Simonton, 1999; Snyder & Pearse, 2010). The family therapist lets the family know that these emotions are normal, expected, and encouraged. Additionally, upon hearing the diagnosis, some family members may be emotionally expressive, while others may remain numb and stoic. These family members are assured that emotional expression is manifested in many different ways, and their expressions are to be respected. The family therapist helps family members to process and normalize their emotions, educates them about the emotional and relational changes brought about by the cancer diagnosis, and teaches them new coping strategies (Ruddy & McDaniel, 2013).

Further, some family members may feel guilty about the BCS diagnosis, engage in self-blame for not doing enough, have regrets about past treatment of the BCS before the diagnosis, or feel angry about not being able to prevent the cancer. The family therapist introduces interventions such as reframing and gender-role analysis, which help the family to mitigate these concerns and focus on the health needs of the BCS instead of engaging in self-blame or regret (Corey, 2017; Goldenberg et al., 2017; Ruddy & McDaniel, 2013). Utilizing the strength-focused approach of feminist therapy, the family therapist can help family members move beyond, feelings of blame and regret and identify opportunities to positively redefine the family dynamic, including mending broken relationships and examining and restructuring gender roles to benefit the needs of the BCS (Corey, 2017).

An important assessment tool that can be used in the early phases of family therapy is the genogram. A genogram provides a real-time view of the family constellation. It is useful in understanding the family's medical and psychiatric history and relational dynamics, the evolution of family relationships and experiences, and family values and themes around the breast cancer diagnosis (Meiers et al., 2015). It can be adapted to include all pertinent individuals and systems that impact upon the wellness of the family, including the extended family, the treatment team, employers, teachers, and spiritual leaders. The genogram's analytical value allows the family therapist to better understand where and how to deploy advocacy resources. Further, the process of developing the genogram can be used as a tool to promote feminist therapy principles including exploring gender role biases, using one's voice, power differentials, providing education, and validating emotions (Kosutic et al., 2009).

The genogram has utility in developing a comprehensive treatment plan and allows the family therapist and family members to examine the progression of treatment goals. The family therapist and family members visually map the shared emotional impact of the illness on the family unit and explore the effectiveness of treatment recommendations by examining the barriers and advances experienced by each family member (Souza et al., 2016). For example, when examining family communication patterns, the family therapist outlines how and with whom the family members communicate. The genogram allows the family members to label and visualize the family interactions, explore the historical context of negative familial behaviors such as poor communication, and adopt strategies to improve the presenting issues (McGoldrick, 2016).

Providing support and psychoeducational resources

Strategies outlined in this section detail the importance of support and psychoeducational resources. The therapeutic applications are grounded in feminist therapy and range from employing family and emotional supports to engagement of strength-focused social networks and community organizations.

For BCS, networks of support provide community, resources, and information. Community and social supports are necessary for BCS as these contacts allow them to connect with others and share the effects of breast cancer on their bodies, families, and feelings (Kroenke et al., 2006; Reynolds et al., 1994; Ucok, 2005). Research has found that social support contributes to improved health and lowered mortality rates for BCS (Reynolds et al., 1994). Adversely, researchers found an increase in mortality rates in BCS populations who lacked close relationships or emotional support (Reynolds et al., 1994). These findings highlight BCS need for support from friends, family, and community members.

A number of research studies have emphasized the impact of family support networks on BCS clinical outcomes (Diallo et al., 2019; Muhamad et al., 2011; Rolland et al., 1999; Snyder & Pearse, 2010; Vrontaras, 2018). Snyder and Pearse (2010) reported that young breast cancer survivors relied on their families for several kinds of support. Emotional support included feeling secure, cared for and understood, having family members to talk with about the cancer, and having family members who were physically present. Tangible support included rides to the medical community, childcare, family members preparing meals, providing physical care during chemotherapy, help with housework, and support through diagnosis and recovery. Informational support involved obtaining educational resources, exploring treatment options, consulting with other doctors, and having family members as advocates. Experiential support was connecting with other BCS and listening to their insights, experiences, and stories of survival.

In a related study on family support in cancer survivorship, Muhamad et al. (2011) found that survivors relied on their family for information on survivorship, managing emotions, collaborating in treatment decisions, lifestyle and dietary practices, spiritual issues, and educational interventions. Diallo et al. (2019) reported that both external and family systems resources impacted caregiver stress and health outcomes, directly influencing BCS health outcomes. Radina and Armer (2001) found that BCS with strong family support and healthy coping mechanisms navigated cancer-related stressors more effectively than BCS without similar support systems.

The family therapist encourages survivor and support network engagement which increases BCS and family members opportunities for consciousness raising, a feminist therapy principle that emphasizes solidarity and shared community experiences. The family therapist, as a resource person, also connects the family and BCS with appropriate levels and types of support which might not have been previously accessible. Interventions centered on familial, peer, patient to patient and tangible support, lead to improved mental health and well-being amongst BCS and their families (Reynolds et al., 1994).

In addition to delivering therapy, the family therapist serves as an invaluable resource. Psychoeducational information on the prevalence, course and prognosis of breast cancer, developmental issues and challenges at each stage of treatment, teaching the family how to work as a team to manage the illness and how to access community resources, are examples of informational resources that a family therapist provides (Diallo et al., 2019; Goldenberg et al., 2017; Rolland et al., 1999). These resources are especially beneficial when working with underserved families who may not have access to this information or have misconceptions about cancer treatment and recovery (Sherman & Simonton, 1999). Additionally, BCS and family members may not understand directives provided by medical staff because these professionals may have limited time, or there may be other existing barriers (e.g., communication, cultural, educational) that prevent full engagement. Providing psychoeducation to empower families creates avenues for advocacy, which is a key component of feminist therapy.

BCS and their family must remain involved and educated about all phases of treatment. Encouraging the family to collaborate with BCS primary care providers is essential for gleaning correct information about treatment and addressing misconceptions about cancer and recovery, including palliative care (Ruddy & McDaniel, 2013). The family therapist serves as a liaison between the family and medical providers, as the family may feel lost, confused, and overwhelmed by the medical systems of care. The family therapist provides information and interventions focused on successful coping and empowering techniques designed to mitigate the family's stress and strain. By creating avenues for information sharing and advocacy surrounding medical treatment, the family therapist gives the family a voice.

Educating family members about respecting BCS boundaries is necessary. Some families may want to cling; others may want to disengage; BCS may want neither, nor to be treated as "sick." BCS may experience stress and frustration when well-meaning family members intervene in every aspect of their daily life and also guilt and confusion because the family is trying to help. Seeking solitude is just as important as family support; a balance of both is necessary for BCS. A breast cancer diagnosis does not take away BCS autonomy, as their voices are valued. The family therapist reminds the family that the diagnosis is not the primary focus and gives them permission to reengage in their pre-cancer lives.

Family members benefit from the information provided by the American Cancer Society, the National Cancer Institute and many other organizations and networks on statistics, symptoms, experiences, and lifestyle changes of BCS and their families. Referral of family members to breast cancer support groups and organizations, religious and spiritual assemblies, and other outside entities focused on cancer treatment and support, provides additional avenues of relief that the family therapist recommends (Sherman & Simonton, 1999). Electronic media, the internet, print media such as newsletters, books, magazines, and brochures, and educational intervention programs based on the needs of the BCS and their families are beneficial for education, learning, outreach, compliance, and clinical outcomes (Muhamad et al., 2011). By encouraging engagement with larger social networks and diverse media platforms, the family therapist supports the BCS in cultivating an enhanced quality of life.

Communication skills and strategies

Effective communication enhances coping, family collaboration, and emotional support (Ruddy & McDaniel, 2013). This section provides guidance to help the family therapist facilitate healthy communication between the BCS and family.

Engaged communication between family members is a treatment goal that the family therapist fosters. A lack of communication and understanding leads to a misinformed diagnosis that harms the BCS and the family and impacts life expectancy outcomes. Open communication within family systems during a breast cancer diagnosis is a challenge for family members. If the information is communicated sensitively, it allows family members to more readily accept the diagnosis, communicate their psychological distress in a safe place, and voice their concerns about the expected family changes and challenges (Rolland et al., 1999; Ruddy & McDaniel, 2013; Sherman & Simonton, 1999).

Rolland et al. (1999) point out that genuine communication during an illness may be hindered by worries about hurting the person, making the condition worse, fearing that the relationship will not survive, and shameful thoughts and feelings. Open communication acknowledges these different perspectives and serves as a conduit for more effective problem solving, family coping, control where there was none, shared responsibility for healing, working collaboratively toward informed decision-making during treatment, and providing needed emotional support (Rolland et al., 1999; Ruddy & McDaniel, 2013; Sherman & Simonton, 1999). The family therapist intervenes and helps the family normalize and process their ambivalence, fear, anger, resentment, helplessness, existential anxiety, and uncertainty; not doing so jeopardizes treatment outcomes for the BCS and for the family.

The delivery of a breast cancer diagnosis to the family must be relayed carefully and thoughtfully. Facilitating meetings where open-ended questions allow for family members to share their reactions to the diagnosis, communicate their angst, and share their thoughts and feelings is an important therapeutic goal. The family therapist can expect an emotional initial counseling session as family members attempt to navigate each other's responses.

Motivating the family to engage in further therapy is a significant intervention, as emotional challenges are likely to continue. Feelings of discouragement, helplessness, and anxiety can be analyzed and processed with continued family therapy to reduce family members' feelings of isolation and disconnect, as well as to engender closer relationships (Sherman & Simonton, 1999).

The family therapist helps the family to communicate with the many medical systems utilized in navigating treatment for the BCS and incorporates feminist therapy principles to carefully examine the personal and political implications of the breast cancer diagnosis. By addressing personal desires and societal expectations of femininity, the family therapist empowers the BCS and family to define the parameters of treatment. The BCS must be a central part of all discussions and decisions. The family therapist also develops collaborative relationships with the interlocking caregiving systems and serves as an advocate for the family and the BCS. For example, if there is a lack of clarity about treatment, the family therapist helps the family to formulate questions about treatment benefits, recommendations, and outcomes. The family therapist does not give advice about medical treatment; instead, the family has the responsibility for decision-making, which enhances their sense of control and mastery of the situation (Ruddy & McDaniel, 2013).

Structural and organizational challenges and caregiver role strain

A diagnosis of breast cancer disrupts the family organization and equilibrium, causes adjustments in familial roles and increases caregiver stress. This section focuses on structural and organizational challenges and caregiver role strain for BCS and their families.

The mental, physical, and financial impact of breast cancer realigns the family's boundaries, hierarchy, subsystems, and organizational structure. There are also role changes, such as the delegation of new and different tasks as well as increased caregiver responsibilities (Diallo et al., 2019; Millington & Madden, 2015). Stenberg et al. (2010) reviewed 192 articles on the effects of caring for a patient with cancer. Over 200 problems and burdens were identified and categorized into physical health problems, financial difficulties, emotional problems, social problems, and burdens related to responsibilities and impact on daily life. The researchers found that family caregivers experience challenging burdens and responsibilities that impacted their effective functioning; therefore, they must be included in patient-care outcomes.

Northouse et al. (2010) conducted a meta-analysis of 29 randomized clinical trials published between 1983–2009, which focused on interventions with family caregivers of cancer patients. The types of interventions offered were psychoeducational, skills training, and therapeutic counseling. Although the interventions had small to medium effects, they were shown to reduce caregiver stress, increase effective coping and self-efficacy, and enhance caregiver quality of life. The researchers concluded that family caregivers' psychosocial needs must be addressed to maintain their health while caring for cancer patients. In a related study by Li et al. (2018), results indicated that despite experiencing a variety of burdens, family resilience helped to promote BCS individual resilience and eased caregiver burden.

Based on the above studies, the family therapist is positioned to engage the family in conversations about role changes, including routines and caregiving responsibilities brought about by the diagnosis. The family therapist can discuss feminist therapy interventions such as gender role analysis, that encourage family caregivers to explore existing constructs of gender, balance responsibilities, and adjust tasks so that the caregiver is not overwhelmed.

Additionally, partners and children are subject to a reversal of roles and responsibilities within the home, as the BCS can no longer complete tasks and responsibilities for herself or her family members (Campbell-Enns & Woodgate, 2017). BCS may feel guilty and conflicted about their decreased capacity to perform their roles as mothers and caregivers while trying to adhere to medical guidelines (Radina & Armer, 2001). Encouraging role flexibility, task modification, maintaining a balance between family and medical needs, and strengthening family structures to reduce stress, are helpful interventions the family therapist can suggest to promote BCS autonomy and contribution to family functioning. These interventions support the feminist therapy principles of resocialization of roles and analysis of power distribution within the family.

To develop useful interventions, the family therapist must understand that the breast cancer diagnosis is a shared experience between the BCS and the family caregiver. As a result, family caregiver resilience, delineated by the caregiver's ability to manage and recover from distress, is directly linked to the BCS resilience. Likewise, resilience, for both the family caregiver and the BCS is also correlated with caregiver burden. Some level of caregiver burden or distress is expected as a result of the breast cancer diagnosis. However, the distress can also be influenced by the age, mental health, financial concerns, and the level of familial support for the BCS and family caregiver (Li et al., 2018).

Interventions that decrease family caregiver distress such as mental health therapy and psychoeducation modalities that focus on improving the caregiver's emotional wellness and coping resources are recommended (Northouse et al., 2010). Further, feminist therapy interventions that reframe caregiver role expectations increase the caregiver's ability to support the BCS. This reduces physical and psychological distress for both the BCS and family caregiver. Additionally, Stenberg et al. (2010) recommends virtual support found on the internet. Some virtual interventions may include the creation of online peer support groups, telehealth used to deliver individual and family therapy, and psychoeducation through the use of media platforms.

Families coping with breast cancer risk creating parentified children, especially in environments where few support systems are available, the family is single parent, or the older sibling is responsible for taking care of the younger siblings. Additionally, the child or adolescent may feel obligated to assume more parental responsibility. Rolland et al. (1999) cautioned that depending on the trajectory of the illness, considerations for the child or adolescent must include role re-definition, distribution of tasks, role blending, and completion of developmental milestones. The family therapist's conversations with the family about role negotiation and role blending, the meaning of added responsibilities for the child or adolescent, and issues of balance, flexibility, and equal responsibility, provide insights into family functioning (Rolland et al., 1999). Establishing boundaries for caregiving responsibilities and allowing the child or adolescent to engage in age-appropriate activities are strategies the family therapist can suggest to ease the guilt and resentment of being thrust into this untenable role. Helping the family to assist the child or adolescent to develop interventions to mitigate the stress arising from caregiving responsibilities is a goal that the family therapist can also support.

Children and adolescents of parents diagnosed with breast cancer are also at increased risks for adverse psychological outcomes. To combat this, families often attempt to insulate children and adolescents from the realities of breast cancer by masking or denying the presenting symptoms and effects of chemotherapy. Further, the adult family members may project positivity, carefully manage information, and hide their emotional distress to divert the children's attention away from the illness (Asbury et al., 2014). However, avoiding difficult conversations about the prognosis and potential impact of breast cancer on the family is not recommended. Despite attempts to shield children and adolescents from the breast cancer diagnosis, they will likely identify cancer-related changes and recognize that something is wrong before being told (Forrest et al., 2006). Kennedy and Lloyd-Williams (2009) explain that children and adolescents want information about breast cancer but resist asking questions to avoid upsetting their parents. The therapist educates the family about communicating the breast cancer diagnosis in an age-appropriate manner and allows children and adolescents to ask questions and express their feelings. This action communicates that their voices and feelings are valued, which is an important feminist therapy principle.

Children and adolescents may be more comfortable discussing their angst with their peers and benefit from supportive peer to peer communication that helps them to balance feelings of isolation and adapt to familial changes resulting from the breast cancer diagnosis (Davey et al., 2005; Ellis et al., 2016). Additionally, children and adolescents benefit from supportive adult relationships that help to maintain predictability and healthy routines. Consistent connection with counselors, teachers, and other family members with whom they feel safe communicating is valuable in facilitating emotional wellness. These adults can aid in providing age-appropriate information regarding the diagnosis, treatment, and prognosis (Kennedy & Lloyd-Williams, 2009). The family therapist can utilize these individuals as additional resources.

The family therapist also implements interventions to help the family members and BCS create and maintain functional relationships within the household. By teaching the family how to adopt strength-focused interventions that reformulate the illness, the family therapist promotes healthy relationship interactions, coping strategies, and flexibility of roles. As a result, BCS experience improved health outcomes (Diallo et al., 2019; Radina & Armer, 2001).

Existential concerns, grieving losses, and family self-care

End-of-life planning is often a difficult and emotionally painful part of cancer treatment.

BCS and their family members often struggle with transitioning from intensive, aggressive treatments to palliation (Gaeta & Price, 2010). This section describes strategies to address the end of curative treatments, manage the challenges of grief and loss, and engage in family self-care.

The family therapist coordinates multidisciplinary treatment team meetings to discuss family roles, prognosis, as well as palliative requests related to the end life process (Gaeta & Price, 2010). Family interaction with the multidisciplinary team fosters rapport building, specifically related to building trust and enhancing communication between the family and the medical team. Feminist therapy interventions that support informed decision-making give voice to the BCS and family and empower them to take ownership of end of life decisions. The family therapist plays a crucial role in supporting families as they navigate these difficult existential issues. These must be handled with sensitivity as families may not be willing or ready to broach the topic (Ruddy & McDaniel, 2013). Additional discussions could include expectations about death, funeral wishes, advanced and living wills, hospice placement, and how to spend remaining time left together (Sherman & Simonton, 1999).

A cancer diagnosis does not mean that the family should stop living, as self-care is the act of preserving oneself and is essential for navigating acute illness and its associated symptoms. The family therapist reinforces feminist principles that reformulate the family's identity by encouraging them to engage in pre-cancer diagnosis activities. Interactions that foster familial connectivity, such as going to the movies and out to dinner, taking trips, engaging in hobbies, and participating in family traditions and spiritual rituals help maintain a sense of normalcy for the family (Ng et al., 2017; Sherman & Simonton, 1999). These activities must include the BCS, as the focus is on providing structure and consistency by staying engaged in everyday living.

Familial relationships are essential for BCS; however, the location where BCS and family members gather is valuable. Årestedt et al. (2016) believe that safe spaces possess rejuvenating components of wellness. For BCS and their families, being inside the home and in other designated homelike spaces is meaningful. A sense of at-homeness allows BCS and their family members to fellowship in a safe space, express their feelings, discuss the breast cancer diagnosis, and regain control over this aspect of their lives. The family therapist can ask family members to create a communal and a private safe space where they can relieve stress, enjoy solitude, and foster family cohesiveness. Both spaces serve different purposes. The construct of at-homeness reflects feminist therapy principles, as it allows the BCS and family members to reframe their sense of home such that it creates feelings of empowerment and healing.

The family therapist can also encourage family members to engage in activities such as exercising, journaling, writing and self-reflection, relaxation techniques, alternate breathing, and progressive muscle relaxation (Karimi et al., 2017; Weingarten & Worthen, 2018). These interventions help to improve their minds, bodies, and spirit and allow the families to focus on their strengths, to problem solve, and to develop alternative healing practices and strategies (Weingarten & Worthen, 2018). The next section includes a brief discussion of mind-body interventions and self-care strategies from which family members and BCS can benefit.

Mind body and expressive art interventions

Families experiencing cancer face transitions that require unique and collaborative approaches to treatment. The adaptability of feminist therapy allows the incorporation of a variety of educational, empowering, and strength-based techniques (Corey, 2017), which can include mind-body interventions. Mind-body interventions such as yoga and tai chi lower symptoms of anxiety and depression through breathing and meditation and are useful in working with BCS and their families (Elkins et al., 2010).

Expressive modalities, such as art, poetry, and music are helpful with BCS and family members when words fail to convey their concerns or fears regarding the diagnosis, their uncertainty about the future, and how to assist the BCS through treatment and recovery.

Expressive arts interventions are strength-focused, deepen understanding of family interactions, and allow the family therapist to identify strengths that the unit currently possesses. What follows is a brief discussion of mind-body techniques and expressive arts interventions that can be utilized with families of BCS.

Mindfulness

Mindfulness based stress reduction (MBSR) has shown effectiveness with mood and emotionally instability, increased stress, poor concentration and strained family relationships, common concerns that family members of BCS may experience (Gambrel & Keeling, 2010; Ngamkham et al., 2019). In a review of mindfulness interventions, Ngamkham et al. (2019), found that out of 1,800 participants, 45% reported experiencing severe family anxiety, further solidifying the need for familial involvement in treatment.

Yoga

Yoga has been utilized as a non-cognitive tool in cancer patient and survivor studies, has proven to be effective in enhancing mental and physical wellness, and is a helpful component in increasing self-awareness in BCS (Milbury et al., 2018). Subedi (2014) discovered that yoga is useful for strengthening interactions and communication with families of BCS. The Stanford Supportive Care Program, sought to improve the quality of life of individuals diagnosed with cancer and their families through yoga. Research findings revealed that these practices improved the general wellbeing of BCS (Rosenbaum et al., 2004). In their review of yoga as an intervention, Danhauer et al. (2017) reported that familial participation in yoga had the potential to improve the overall health of the caregivers. Mackenzie et al. (2016) reported benefits linked to the use of yoga among cancer caregivers. They included normalization of cancer centered discussions, alternate worldviews of the disease, a decrease in stress, and feeling less burdened. In a couples based Tibetan yoga program for lung cancer patients, caregivers experienced a decrease in fatigue and anxiety and had fewer sleep disturbances (Milbury et al., 2015).

Although yoga has been found to increase mind-body connections, more research is needed to measure its success in family therapy. The utilization of feminist therapy and yoga in an individual or group setting allows for reframing. Family therapists can incorporate the feminist therapy interventions of reframing and empowerment when BCS and their family members engage in yoga. This allows BCS and their family members to reflect upon their own experiences with the disease and create an uplifting narrative which focuses on positive outcomes.

Tai Chi

Similar to yoga, engagement in tai chi yields significant diminution in anxiety and depression and an increase in relaxation, uninterrupted sleep, and social support, all of which are beneficial to families and BCS as they seek healthy ways to navigate the challenges of breast cancer (Galantino et al., 2013). Tai Chi is a slow form of martial arts that employs deep breathing, continuous deliberate movements, relaxation techniques, and standing meditation, which are designed to increase balance and strength and promote well-being (Galantino et al., 2013). Both yoga and Tia Chi increase family socialization, interactions, and mutual support needed during a breast cancer diagnosis and treatment (Galantino et al., 2013).

Art

Art therapy with the family aids in identifying gender roles, power differentials, and reframing maladaptive thinking among family members (Malchiodi, 2007). Art has been a long-standing medium for personal expression. Studies indicate that art therapy is an effective strategy for reducing pain and improving the overall wellness and survival of cancer patients (Pelletier, 2004; Stanczyk, 2011). Art is not only limited to reducing stress but can also produce heightened awareness through self-exploration and give a voice to family members who may be unable or too intimidated to express themselves accurately or emotionally (Malchiodi, 2007).

Interventions such as Mandala art therapy help individuals to communicate suppressed emotions (Malchiodi, 2007). When interpreted, repressed feelings may emerge, uncovering concerns surrounding gender role analysis and power differentials. For example, the BCS may experience difficulty with loss of breasts, loss of femininity, and loss of power as a woman. Further, through art, the family therapist gains insight into family communication patterns and perspectives of the breast cancer diagnosis (Malchiodi, 2007).

Poetry

Poetry is another useful form of creative expression. Written expression assists in the success of physical and emotional recovery, allows for an intimate exploration of the experience and gives clarity to family therapists regarding family concerns (Malchiodi, 2007). Through the lens of feminist therapy, poetry as a treatment modality illustrates personal political undertones (e.g., health care disparities, discrimination, limited economic resources) that promote a commitment to social change and gives credence to the family's struggles related to the breast cancer diagnosis. The use of poetry ties into the tenet of women's voices being heard and honored through written expression. It provides strength-based avenues for reframing experiences and reconnecting with self (Reilly et al., 2018). Reframing can be utilized in family therapy sessions with BCS, as it allows family members to reimagine the diagnosis into something more positive to facilitate change. As with art therapy, poetry can be used with family members to open closed doors of communication.

Music

Research indicates that music is beneficial in decreasing anxiety, depression, mood disturbances, and pain related to cancer (Carlson et al., 2017; Elkins et al., 2010). Music can evoke strong emotions and thoughts through its melodic and rhythmic charm. It inspires and validates feelings of power and hope and has been found useful in treating cancer patients and their families (Carlson et al., 2017). For example, family members who are not overly emotional can be asked to express their feelings through music selection (e.g., jazz, rock, gospel, hip-hop, country) or music lyrics. Similarly, family members who are numb from the impact of the breast cancer diagnosis or who cannot identify their feelings may be able to do so through musical expression. By encouraging the family unit to engage in musical expression, family therapists support BCS and their families in allowing diverse voices to be heard.

Implications for practice

A breast cancer diagnosis is devastating and creates burdens for BCS and their families. Family therapy interventions help to mitigate these stressors. There are several implications for family therapists. First, the extant literature reflects a dominant culture perspective that omits the marginalization and healthcare disparities experienced by underserved populations, including sexual minorities and families of color. Therefore, family therapists must be well versed in continuity of care, family advocacy, and integrative treatment planning that addresses the biopsychosocial and cultural needs of diverse families of BCS. Integrative treatment practices should become the standard of care to prevent treatment from becoming exclusive to some BCS families instead of inclusive to all BCS families.

Additionally, cultural competency training to deliver effective clinical care, to understand the obstacles and stressors experienced by underserved families, and to increase the family therapist's toolbox of interventions should be ongoing. Finally, family therapists must lend their voices to individual, group, institutional, and societal advocacy initiatives that focus on robust national policies that support families in crisis. They can work to remove external barriers that prevent families of BCS from accessing needed resources. Therapists can develop curriculum materials and academic resources that address these underserved families. They can engage in community campaigns, healthcare initiatives, and partnerships that address the needs of families of BCS. These initiatives help to improve the quality of life of both the families and BCS.

Limitations and future research

There are several limitations within this manuscript. First, the information is not generalizable to all families of breast cancer survivors, especially those who do not have the resources, time, or the ability to engage in therapy. Research that includes interventions that are helpful to families across all demographics (e.g., socioeconomic status, single, blended, special needs, underserved) is needed because breast cancer does not discriminate.

Further, finding a robust body of research data on interventions for families of breast cancer survivors was challenging. Some data exists in piecemeal fashion instead of in central bodies of work. The paucity of research is surprising, considering that breast cancer is the most frequently occurring cancer among women. Not only is more research needed on this topic, but the data should be easily accessed. Another limitation is that research on this topic reflects a dominant culture family structure orientation (e.g., couples, sound support systems, available resources, dominant culture values, and practices). As a result, the available research largely excludes a broad spectrum of families and does not reflect balanced, inclusive, cultural perspectives.

Finally, the manuscript is not an empirical study; therefore, research utilizing sound methodology and focused on family and caregiver adaptation, the effectiveness of mind-body interventions, and culturally appropriate interventions for families and BCS would benefit the field. Empirical studies provide family therapists with a sound framework for understanding the challenges experienced by families of BCS and give them additional tools to utilize in treatment with families from all demographics.

Conclusion

A breast cancer diagnosis is a monumental challenge fraught with medical and psychosocial uncertainty for BCS and their families. Family therapy offers clinical interventions to address these challenges. Robust research is scant in many areas such as caregiver and family adaptation, families from underserved populations, and appropriate cultural interventions. Family therapists can bridge this gap by providing focused therapeutic services. Family therapists can incorporate gender role analyses, strength-based approaches, reframing, and a recognition of oppressive factors to highlight the unique social and cultural experiences of BCS. Finally, family therapists can incorporate feminist therapy into their practice by recognizing different oppressive factors which historically and contemporarily impact BCS and their families politically and socially (Kosutic et al., 2009). Such services reflect an understanding of the family's issues, promote family strength and resiliency, and model competent, quality, culturally sensitive clinical care while exploring interventions designed to help BCS and their families through a difficult experience.

References

Årestedt, L., Benzein, E., Persson, C., & Rämgård, M. (2016). A shared respite: The meaning of place for family well-being in families living with chronic illness. *International Journal of Qualitative Studies on Health and Well-being, 11*(1), 1–10. https://doi.org/10.3402/qhw.v11.30308

Asbury, N., Lalayiannis, L., & Walshe, A. (2014). How do I tell the children? Women's experiences of sharing information about breast cancer diagnosis and treatment. *European Journal of Oncology Nursing, 18*(6), 564–570. https://doi.org/10.1016/j.ejon.2014.07.003

Campbell-Enns, H., & Woodgate, R. (2017). The psychosocial experiences of women with breast cancer across the lifespan: A systematic review. *Psycho-Oncology, 26*(11), 1711–1721. https://doi.org/10.1002/pon.4281

Carlson, L., Rouleau, C., Speca, M., Robinson, J., & Bultz, B. D. (2017). Brief supportive-expressive group therapy for partners of men with early stage prostate cancer: Lessons learned from a negative randomized controlled trial. *Support Care Cancer, 25*(4), 1035–1041. https://doi.org/10.1007/s00520-016-3551-1

Corey, G. (2017). *Theory and practice of counseling and psychotherapy* (10th ed.). Cengage Learning.

Danhauer, S., Addington, E., Sohl, S., Chaoul, A., & Cohen, L. (2017). Review of yoga therapy during cancer treatment. *Support Care Cancer, 25*(4), 1357–1372. https://doi.org/10.1007/s00520-016-3556-9

Davey, M., Gulish, L., Askew, J., Godette, K., & Childs, N. (2005). Adolescents coping with mom's breast cancer: Developing family intervention programs. *Journal of Marital and Family Therapy, 31*(2), 247–258. https://doi.org/10.1111/j.1752-0606.2005.tb01558.x

Diallo, A., Cuevas, S., Vang, C., & Vemu, S. (2019). Caregiving and stress: Family- systems resources and external resources. *Journal of Rehabilitation, 85*(4) 4–13.

Elkins, G., Fisher, W., & Johnson, A. (2010). Mind–body therapies in integrative oncology. *Current Treatment Options in Oncology, 11*(3–4), 128–140. https://doi.org/10.1007/s11864-010-0129-x

Ellis, S., Wakefield, C., Antill, G., Burns, M., & Patterson, P. (2016). Supporting children facing a parent's cancer diagnosis: A systematic review of children's psychosocial needs and existing interventions. *European Journal of Cancer Care, 1*(26), 22. https://doi.org/10.1111/ecc.12432

Forrest, G., Plumb, C., Ziebland, S., & Stein, A. (2006). Breast cancer in the family: Children's perceptions of their mother's cancer and its initial treatment: Qualitative study. *BMJ, 332* (7548), 998–1003. https://doi.org/10.1136/bmj.38793.567801.AE

Gaeta, S., & Price, K. (2010). End-of-life issues in critically ill cancer patients. *Critical Care Clinics, 26*(1), 219–227. https://doi.org/10.1016/j.ccc.2009.10.002

Galantino, M., Callens, M., Cardena, G., Piela, N., & Mao, J. (2013). Tai chi for the well-being of breast cancer survivors with aromatase inhibitor-associated arthralgias: A feasibility study. *Alternative Therapies, 19*(6), 38–44. http://www.alternative-therapies.com/openaccess/ATHM_19-5_taichai.pdf

Gambrel, L. E., & Keeling, M. L. (2010). Relational aspects of mindfulness: Implications for the practice of and family therapy. *Contemporary Family Therapy, 32*(4), 412–426. https://doi.org/10.1007/s10591marriage-010-9129-z

Goldenberg, H., Stanton, M., & Goldenberg, I. (2017). *Family therapy: An overview.* Cengage Learning.

Karimi, S., Makhsosi, B., Seyedi-Andi, S., Behzadi, M., Moghofeh, Y., Mohammadinasrabadi, K., Abdi, A., & Ahmadi, P. (2017). Surveying the effect of a self-care education program on severity of nausea and emesis in colorectal cancer patients under chemotherapy. *Journal of Multidisciplinary Healthcare, 2010*(10), 301–307. https://doi.org/10.2147/JMDH.S131111

Kennedy, V., & Lloyd-Williams, M. (2009). Information and communication when a parent has advanced cancer. *Journal of Affective Disorders, 114*(1–3), 149–155. https://doi.org/10.1016/j.jad.2008.06.022

Kosutic, I., Garcia, M., Graves, T., Barnett, F., Hall, J., Haley, E., Rock, J., Bathon, A., & Kaiser, B. (2009). The critical genogram: A tool for promoting critical consciousness. *Journal of Feminist Family Therapy, 21*(3), 151–176. https://doi.org/10.1080/08952830903079037

Kroenke, C., Kubzansky, L., Schernhammer, E., Holmes, M., & Kawachi, I. (2006). Social networks, social support, and survival after breast cancer diagnosis. *Journal of Clinical Oncology, 24*(7), 1105–1111. https://doi.org/10.1200/JCO.2005.04.2846

Li, Y., Wang, K., Yin, Y., Li, Y., & Li, S. (2018). Relationships between family resilience, breast cancer survivors' individual resilience, and caregiver burden: A cross-sectional study. *International Journal of Nursing Studies, 88*, 79–84. https://doi.org/10.1016/j.ijnurstu.2018.08.011

Mackenzie, M., Wurz, A., Yamauchi, Y., Pires, L., & Culos-Reed, S. (2016). Yoga helps put the pieces back together: A qualitative exploration of a community-based yoga program for cancer survivors. *Evidence-Based Complementary and Alternative Medicine, (2016*, 1–10. https://doi.org/10.1155/2016/1832515

Malchiodi, C. A. (2007). *The art therapy sourcebook*. McGraw-Hill Professional Publishing.

McGoldrick, M. (2016). *The genogram casebook: A clinical companion to genograms: Assessment and intervention*. W.W. Norton & Company.

Meiers, S., Krumwiede, N., Denham, S., & Bell, S. (2015). Family assessment. In S. Denham, P. Eggenberger, N. Young, & N. Krumwiede (Eds.), *Family- focused nursing care* (pp. 1–10). FA Davis.

Milbury, K., Chaoul, A., Engle, R., Liao, Z., Yang, C., Carmack, C., Shannon, V., Spelman, A., Wangyal, T., & Cohen, L. (2015). Couple-based Tibetan yoga program for lung cancer patients and their caregivers. *Psycho-Oncology, 24*(1), 117–120. https://doi.org/https://doi:10.1002/pon.3588

Milbury, K., Mallaiah, S., Mahajan, A., Armstrong, T., Weathers, S. P., Moss, K., Goktepe, N., Spelman, A., & Cohen, L. (2018). Yoga program for high-grade glioma patients undergoing radiotherapy and their family caregivers. *Integrative Cancer Therapies, 17*(2), 332–336. https://doi.org/10.1177/1534735417689882

Millington, M., & Madden, R. (2015). Counseling in the context of family identity. In M. J. Millington & I. Marini (Eds.), *Families in rehabilitation counseling* (pp. 21–46). Springer.

Mitschke, D. B. (2008). Cancer in the family: Review of the psychosocial perspectives of patients and family members. *Journal of Family Social Work, 11*(2), 166–184. https://doi.org/10.1080/10522150802175159

Muhamad, M., Afshari, M., & Kazilan, F. (2011). Family support in cancer survivorship. *Asian Pacific Journal of Cancer Prevention, 12*(6), 1389–1397.

Ng, Z., Ong, M., Jegadeesan, T., Deng, S., & Yap, C. (2017). Breast cancer: Exploring the facts and holistic needs during and beyond treatment. *Healthcare, 5*(2), 26. https://doi.org/10.3390/healthcare5020026

Ngamkham, S., Holden, J., & Smith, E. L. (2019). A systematic review: Mindfulness intervention for cancer-related pain. *Asia-Pacific Journal of Oncology Nursing, 6*(2), 161–169. https://doi.org/10.4103/apjon.apjon_67_18

Northouse, L., Katapodi, M., Song, L., Zhang, L., & Mood, D. W. (2010). Interventions with family caregivers of cancer patients: Meta-analysis of randomized trials. *CA: A Cancer Journal for Clinicians*, 60(5), 317–339. https://doi.org/10.3322/caac.20081

Pelletier, C. (2004). The effect of music on decreasing arousal due to stress: A meta- analysis. *Journal of Music Therapy*, 41(3), 192–214. https://doi.org/10.1093/jmt/41.3.192

Radina, M., & Armer, J. (2001). Post-breast cancer lymphedema and the family: A qualitative investigation of families coping with chronic illness. *Journal of Family Nursing*, 7(3), 281–299. https://doi.org/10.1177/107484070100700305

Reilly, R., Lee, V., Laux, K., & Robitaille, A. (2018). Using found poetry to illuminate the existential and post traumatic growth of women with breast cancer engaging in art therapy. *Qualitative Research in Psychology*, 15(2–3), 196–217. https://doi.org/10.1080/14780887.2018.1429863

Reynolds, P., Boyd, P., Blacklow, R., Jackson, J., Greenberg, R., Austin, D., Bransfield, D., Chen, V., Muss, H., Wesley, M., Hankey, B., Forman, M., Eley, J., Flanders, D., & Edwards, B. (1994). The relationship between social ties and survival among black and white breast cancer patients. National cancer institute black/white cancer survival study group. *Cancer Epidemiology Biomarkers & Prevention*, 3(3), 253–259. https://doi.org/10.1177/107484070100700305

Rolland, J., Altschuler, J., & McFadyen, A. (1999). Parental illness and disability: A family systems framework. *Special Issue: Parental Illness. Journal of Family Therapy*, 21(3), 242. https://doi.org/10.1111/1467-6427.00118.

Rosenbaum, E., Gautier, H., Fobair, P., Neri, E., Festa, B., Hawn, M., Andrews, A., Hirshberger, N., Selim, S., & Spiegel, D. (2004). Cancer supportive care, improving the quality of life for cancer patients. A program evaluation report. *Support Care Cancer*, 12(5), 293–301. https://doi.org/10.1007/s00520-004-0599-0

Ruddy, N., & McDaniel, S. (2013). Medical family therapy in the age of health care reform. *Couple and Family Psychology: Research and Practice*, 2(3), 179–191. https://doi.org/10.1037/cfp0000010

Sherman, A., & Simonton, S. (1999). Family therapy for cancer patients: Clinical issues and interventions. *The Family Journal*, 7(1), 39–50. https://doi.org/10.1177/1066480799071006

Snyder, K., & Pearse, W. (2010). Crisis, social support, and the family response: Exploring the narratives of young breast cancer survivors. *Journal of Psychosocial Oncology*, 28(4), 413–431. https://doi.org/10.1080/07347332.2010.484830

Souza, Í., Bellato, R., Araújo, L., & Almeida, K. (2016). Genogram and Eco-map as tools for understanding family care in chronic illness of the young. *Texto & Contexto-Enfermagem*, 25(4), 10. https://doi.org/10.1590/0104-07072016001530015

Stanczyk, M. (2011). Music therapy in supportive cancer care. *Reports of Practical Oncology & Radiotherapy*, 16(5), 170–172. https://doi.org/10.1016/j.rpor.2011.04.005

Stenberg, U., Ruland, C., & Miaskowski, C. (2010). Review of the literature on the effects of caring for a patient with cancer. *Psycho-oncology*, 19(10), 1013–1025. https://doi.org/10.1002/pon.1670

Subedi, S. (2014). Exploring different types of hatha yoga for patients with cancer. *Clinical Journal of Oncology Nursing*, 18(5), 586–590. https://doi.org/10.1188/14.CJON.586-590

Ucok, O. (2005). The meaning of appearance in surviving breast cancer. *Human Studies*, 28(3), 291–316. https://doi.org/10.1007/s10746-005-7412-z

Vrontaras, N. (2018). Cancer patients' views on the family changes and the family social support. *Journal of European Psychology Students*, 9(1), 16–27. https://doi.org/10.5334/jeps.403

Weingarten, K., & Worthen, M. (2018). The solace of an uncertain future: Acute illness, the self, and self-care. *Family Process*, 57(2), 572–586. https://doi.org/10.1111/famp.12347

Relationship of Optimism, Pessimism, and Dysfunctional Career Thoughts in Breast Cancer Survivors from the Bahamas

Levette S. Scott ⓘ, Carlos P. Zalaquett, Herbert Exum, Jeffrey D. Kromrey, Cheryl R. Ellerbrock, and Raheem J. Paxton ⓘ

ABSTRACT
A breast cancer diagnosis can lead to life-altering biopsychosocial changes and challenges for breast cancer survivors (BCS). Particularly salient is body image perception and its associated biopsychosocial ramifications. This manuscript examined the impact of breast cancer on women's body image, including women of color and lesbians. The information was contextualized through the application of feminist theory principles. Interventions and implications for breast cancer survivors (BCS) were discussed utilizing feminist theory.

The American Cancer Society identifies breast cancer as the most frequently diagnosed cancer in women. In 2019, approximately 268,600 women will be diagnosed, and 41,760 will die from the disease (American Cancer Society, 2019). Though White women are diagnosed at higher rates, 42% more Black women die of breast cancer compared to White women (Foy et al., 2018). The Centers for Disease Control Prevention's 2016 snapshot of the breast cancer mortality rates among the U.S. female demographic indicates that per 100,000 cases, approximately 27% Black, 20% White, 14% Latina, 12% American Indian/Alaska Native, and 11% Asian/Pacific Islander women in the country die of breast cancer (Center for Disease Control and Prevention, 2016)

A diagnosis of breast cancer has pervasive consequences on a woman's physical and mental health. The breasts signal femininity and are physical emblems of womanhood. However, breast cancer and the associated treatments such as surgery, chemotherapy, and adjunctive hormone therapy, leave a woman physically and psychologically ravaged. The effects of scarring, breast and hair loss, and reduced sexual and reproductive functioning leave her to grapple with issues of body image and previously held ideas of sexuality, femininity, and wholeness as a woman (Boquiren et al., 2013). For this manuscript, data on breast cancer, body image, and their impact on breast cancer survivors (BCS), including the family, are presented and contextualized through the application of feminist theory principles and interventions. Implications for BCS are discussed.

A theoretical framework for understanding breast cancer and body image

Several theories provide a framework for understanding body image difficulties among BCS. The cognitive behavioral model of body image purported by Cash (2011) includes body image evaluation and body image investment. Body image evaluation refers to the degree of satisfaction with one's body and any discrepancies between the real and ideal physical self-image, while body image investment encapsulates the overall physical appearance. Another cognitive behavioral model by White (2002) emphasizes survivor perceptions and experiences of appearance changes, whether those changes are noticeable or not. Changes from breast cancer will result in negative body image depending on the level of body investment and any discrepancy between the real and ideal physical self-image. Fingeret et al. (2013) theoretical framework place body image concerns of BCS on a continuum ranging from mild to extreme. Survivors with more pronounced body image concerns interact less favorably with others and BCS minimize body image difficulties because of shame or embarrassment (Fingeret et al., 2013).

Conceptually, body image includes perceptions, thoughts, feelings, and behaviors related to the body's appearance, functions, and capabilities (Fingeret et al., 2014; Paterson et al., 2016). Negative body image creates lifelong challenges that impact a survivor's recovery. Disease and treatment fallout include appearance alterations, sensory changes, functional impairments, exacerbation of menopausal symptoms, and threats to reproductive capacity (Lewis-Smith et al., 2018). These challenges increase a survivor's psychological vulnerability and result in a plethora of clinical outcomes.

The empirical literature on body image and BCS reveals mixed findings. Researchers have linked a positive body image with increased coping skills, but also reported BCS negative perceptions such as displeasure and insecurity with personal appearance, loss of femininity, physical incompleteness, unwillingness to view their naked form, decreased attractiveness, and discontent with surgical scarring (Pikler & Winterowd, 2003). In other studies, BCS experienced altered views of their bodies and felt less attractive and more disfigured following treatment (Paterson et al., 2016; Van Puymbroeck et al., 2011).

Body image is a very salient concern for younger BCS, and many of the issues with which they struggle involve loss of breasts following surgery (Paterson et al., 2016). The National Cancer Institute estimated that 33% of new breast cancer diagnoses were in women 54 years or younger (Howard-Anderson et al., 2012). Results from a systematic review of 36 body image studies published from 2000–2014 and including 9,343 participants, indicated

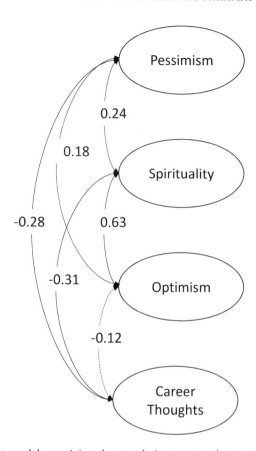

Figure 1. Measurement model examining the correlations among latent constructs. This model was a close fit to the data (2= 59.3, DF=48, RMSEA = 0.03, CFI =0.98, SRMR = 0.04). Solid lines represent statistically significant relationships, whereas dashed lines represent non-significant relationships.

that younger BCS experienced poorer body image, psychological and physical distress, poorer global health, sexuality and intimacy issues, and poor partnered relationships (Paterson et al., 2016). The researchers concluded that this population's vulnerability to negative treatment effects and aggressive cancers underscores the urgency of developing empirically sound interventions to address body image disturbance.

A related review (Fingeret et al., 2014) included 92 studies published from 2003–2013 on body image difficulties. Findings specific to BCS included increased body image concerns, adverse psychological stress, higher levels of anxiety and depression, lower quality of life, and poorer sexual functioning. Similarly, Rezaei et al. (2016) reviewed 44 published studies from 1993–2016 on factors influencing body image of BCS. The researchers identified bio-psycho-economic, treatment, disease, physical appearance, and sexual functioning factors as impacting BCS psychological functioning and body image.

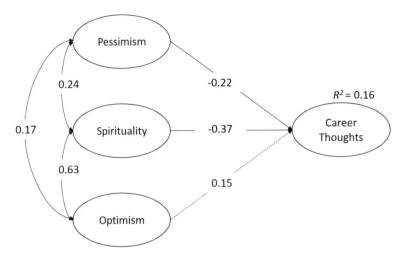

Figure 2. Initial structural model depicting direct linear relationships between pessimism, spirituality, and optimism with careerthoughts. This model was a close fit to the data (2= 59.3, DF=48, RMSEA = 0.03, CFI = 0.98, SRMR = 0.04). Unidirectionalarrows represent linear path coefficients, whereas bidirectional arrows represent correlation among constructs. All coefficientswere standardized. Solid lines represent statistically significant relationships, whereas dashed lines represent non-significantrelationships.

Researchers also investigated gender socialization and body consciousness on body image disturbance in BCS (Boquiren et al., 2013). They found that BCS who internalized traditional gender roles and attitudes experienced greater body shame and body image disturbance and a poorer quality of life. Similarly, in a study of the quality of life of BCS 4 to 42 months after diagnosis, researchers concluded that younger BCS risk an impaired quality of life for several years after diagnosis (Avis et al., 2005). In another longitudinal study on body image and psychosocial adjustment, Moreira and Canavarro (2010) found that having a mastectomy was associated with shame and lower appearance satisfaction, and initial body image did not affect later body image appearance in BCS.

The literature reviewed substantiated that body image is associated with a variety of adverse outcomes for BCS. It emphasized the need for further research to address negative body image concerns and to design new treatment modalities. Also, methodological issues such as small sample sizes, limited diversity of participants, and variations in assessment tools and research designs (Fingeret et al., 2014; Paterson et al., 2016) impacted the generalizability of the findings.

Biopsychosocial challenges for breast cancer survivors

In addition to body image, BCS struggle with other biopsychosocial issues that affect their diagnosis and treatment. The ramifications place additional stress

Table 1 Descriptive Characteristics of Study Participants (n=212)

	n (%)
Age group (n=1 missing)	
18-49 years	88 (42%)
50-59 years	76 (36%)
60+ years	47 (22%)
Education (n=3 missing)	
High school or less	100 (48%)
Some college or more	109 (52%)
Married (n=1 missing)	110 (52%)
Years out from (n=1 missing)	
1-2 years	57 (27%)
3-4 years	32 (15%)
5+ years	122 (58%)
Disease stage at diagnosis (n=24 missing)	
Stage I	95 (51%)
Stage II	49 (26%)
Stage III +	44 (23%)
Pre-cancer employment (n=1 missing)	189 (90%)
Current employment (n=)	111 (53%)

on BCS and compound an already complex situation. Challenges include financial, physical, sexual, social, and clinical concerns.

Financial instability directly impacts BCS ability to access quality care as well as their survival rates. The loss of economic viability combined with the medical expenses of a breast cancer diagnosis affects not only the BCS but also family members and partners (Rotter et al., 2018). Financial stability is essential for the purposes of extended medical stays, procedures, medications, and co-pays. It is helpful for BCS to have the support of spousal finances and insurance to avoid financial strain. Financial instability is especially taxing on BCS because of the economic hardship, financial distress, and financial burden it causes (Ashing et al., 2018). Insurance concerns and directives present additional obstacles, primarily since levels of coverage differ, health care plans vary, and some BCS cannot afford treatment without insurance (Rotter et al., 2018). Findings from a study on patient recommendations for reducing the financial burden after breast cancer included expansion of insurance and insurance covered items, domestic and financial assistance from diagnosis through treatment, and preserving previous employment (Dean et al., 2019).

BCS also experience a variety of physical changes stemming from breast loss. Resulting concerns include hormone imbalances, hair loss, fluctuations in weight, the development of adjuvant tumors, scarring and disfiguration, nerve damage, and unfavorable skin color changes resulting from chemotherapy and radiation (Boquiren et al., 2013; Lewis-Smith et al., 2018). Research on body image and BCS and the disease and treatment process confirm the above findings (Fingeret et al., 2014; Rezaei et al., 2016). These changes lead to frequent medical crises and uncertainty about surviving.

Table 2 Associations between Study Covariates and Relevant Latent Constructs

	Career Thoughts	Spirituality	Pessimism	Optimism
Current employment	-0.28*	-0.27	-0.28	-0.09
Education	0.15	-0.35*	0.15	-0.33*
Marital Status	-0.37**	-0.03	0.09	0.04
Pre-cancer employment	-0.51	-0.73*	-0.59*	0.04

Note. * P < 0.05, ** P < 0.01

Struggles with sexuality also plague BCS. In a study of body image and sexual problems in 549 BCS aged 22–50, difficulties related to sexuality, sexual activity, early menopause, body image and physical appearance, poorer mental health, and lack of partners understanding of BCS feelings were reported (Fobair & Spiegel, 2009; Fobair et al., 2006). Related research found that increased preoccupation with body image in younger BCS makes them more amenable to breast reconstruction (Paterson et al., 2016). A relevant study of 90 younger BCS found that those who had mastectomies reported poor sexual functioning, depression, and lower body image than those in the mastectomy reconstruction and control groups (Archangelo et al., 2019).

Nineteen studies on sexual dysfunction published from 2002–2017 were systematically reviewed (Jing et al., 2019) including 2,684 BCS who were administered a brief self-report measure of female sexual function. The researchers reported that women with breast cancer had higher female sexual dysfunction prevalence rates and lower sexual function, and American women with breast cancer had average female sexual dysfunction prevalence and lower average sexual function than Asian women with breast cancer (Jing et al., 2019).

Findings from other studies indicated that BCS in partnered relationships remain sexually active while receiving treatment for their breast cancer; however, many women opt out of sexual encounters, as they are prone to experiencing difficulties with sexual activity, performance, and physical appearance (Fobair et al., 2006; Oberguggenberger et al., 2017). For women in partnered relationships, sexual inadequacy and body unattractiveness inhibited their levels of intimacy and comfort with their sexuality. BCS also struggled with dating, keeping their breast cancer diagnosis a secret, and termination of or change in a partnered relationship (Trachtenberg, 2012).

Social relationships and role strain factors cause additional distress. Protective factors for BCS include family, friends, supportive networks, groups, and professional resources (Campbell-Enns & Woodgate, 2017). Consequently, if BCS cannot maintain healthy relationships with these communities, it will be difficult for them to adapt to changes brought about by breast cancer. BCS experience alienation from peers who shun them and perceive them as sick because of the fear that accompanies a breast cancer diagnosis (Trachtenberg, 2012). For young BCS, the physical ramifications of treatment create fertility issues (Howard-Anderson et al., 2012). An inability to fulfill maternal tasks has a psychological impact on BCS and reshapes how others view them. Because society associates women with being nurturers who use their breasts for feeding, BCS will feel inadequate if they are unable to execute this role (Boquiren et al., 2013; Inhestern & Bergelt, 2018). For example, a review of 28 articles published from 1990–2010 on quality of life, fertility, and health outcomes in younger breast cancer survivors, indicated that younger BCS experienced more psychosocial and menopausal issues than older BCS. These stressors negatively affected their overall health (Howard-Anderson et al., 2012).

Breast cancer survivors are also at risk for one or more clinical disorders such as post-traumatic stress disorder, depression, anxiety, low self-esteem and self-worth, loneliness, and suicidal ideation (Ashing et al., 2018). BCS most commonly experience depression, which results in a diminished standard of life for one in five BCS (Boing et al., 2019). BCS often fear death, experience a tremendous loss of control, and feel taken prisoner by the illness. Therefore, it is not unusual for BCS to have suicidal thoughts, especially following a mastectomy (Szumacher, 2006). The inability to process the trauma of a breast cancer diagnosis results in emotional dysregulation, frustration, spontaneous emotional outbursts, and mood swings that affect BCS personal, professional, and family relationships (Grecucci et al., 2015).

Women of color and lesbian breast cancer survivors: treatment disparities

It is necessary to understand women of color and lesbian BCS lived experiences. Limited research has indicated that body image concerns are not as critical an issue for women of color BCS because of cultural factors (Ashing-Giwa et al., 2004); however, many of these women have limited economic, physical, social, and psychological resources to aid in their recovery from breast cancer (Ashing et al., 2018). Therefore, they remain underserved and at risk for substandard or no treatment, thereby increasing their mortality rates as confirmed by the Center for Disease Control and Prevention (2016).

Research on women of color and lesbian BCS is limited. Available research outlines a familiar theme, that women of color and lesbian BCS report the poorest results with breast cancer survival rates, body image concerns, and overall psychological distress (Patel-Kerai et al., 2017). Mortality among Black women is more than 40% higher than that of White women, and Black women die from breast cancer due to discontinuation of treatment and late diagnosis (Richardson et al., 2016). Black and Latina women postpone and ignore mammograms and follow up recommendations for a variety of reasons, thus increasing their risk for more severe types of breast cancer and shorter survival rates (Yedjou et al., 2017). Additionally, cultural mores and crises influence these women's decisions to undergo cancer screenings and treatment (Patel-Kerai et al., 2017).

Latina women BCS are ambivalent regarding screenings and follow-up care, feeling that healing comes from God instead of medical technology, and reported difficulties communicating with their medical provider (Ashing-Giwa et al., 2004). Results of a survey of 6,722 BCS of all racial and ethnic backgrounds indicated that 19% reported communication problems with their providers, and of this 19%, White BCS (16%) had fewer problems than Black (23%) and Latina (33%) BCS. Culture also influences who determines the survivor's healthcare decisions, and many providers seemed to have a standardized format for diagnosis and treatment of breast cancer without considering the women's health literacy and cultural beliefs (King et al., 2008).

Research on body image across four racial groups (Black, Asian American, Latina and White) revealed that Black and South Asian BCS stated more body image concerns than White women (Patel-Kerai et al., 2017), which is different from results found by (Ashing-Giwa et al., 2004). Further, women from all groups reported challenges adjusting to physical changes from breast cancer, with White women expressing anger and disappointment for getting breast cancer despite their healthy lifestyle. Frequent comments centered on body disgust, decreased self-worth and attractiveness, feeling deformed and inadequate, and a sense of loss.

Ashing-Giwa et al. (2004) conducted a qualitative study of the breast cancer experiences of Black, White, Asian, and Latina BCS. Results indicated that some Black BCS were unwilling to accept their bodies and feared their partner's rejection of their physical appearance; other Black BCS affirmed that breast cancer did not diminish their roles as women, mothers, or wives. Latina BCS worried about weight gain and self-acceptance, while Asian BCS were distressed by their changed bodies. Self-acceptance was more difficult for younger women, and older women viewed their bodies less negatively (Ashing-Giwa et al., 2004).

Boehmer et al. (2013) suggested that resiliency following treatment is higher in lesbian and bisexual survivors, as these survivors use similar coping strategies to navigate both sexual identity discrimination and survivorship (Boehmer et al., 2013). Lesbian BCS are at an increased risk for breast cancer because of less frequent mammogram screenings than cisgender women (Bazzi et al., 2015), extended use of hormones and delay in childbirth (Szumacher, 2006), reduced pregnancy rates (Quinn et al., 2015), and alcohol use, smoking, and obesity (Meads & Moore, 2013). Meads and Moore (2013) reviewed 198 studies on incidence, prevalence rates, and risk studies on breast cancer in lesbians, and bisexual women, and suggested a lack of clarity about higher incidences of breast cancer among lesbians because of the poor methodological quality of the studies. The authors suggested that collecting sexual orientation data from cancer registries or large cohort studies is best (Meads & Moore, 2013). Although it seems that lesbians and bisexual women have an increased prevalence of breast cancer risk factors, it is unclear if they are indeed at an increased risk of breast cancer (Quinn et al., 2015).

Breast cancer contextualized: application and discussion of feminist principles

Cognitive behavioral interventions, guided imagery, psychosexual therapy, cosmetic interventions, massage therapy, yoga, and exercise are cited as interventions for targeting the body image distress of BCS (Fingeret et al., 2014; Lewis-Smith et al., 2018). However, understanding the socio-political context of BCS distress provides additional information about their experiences. Feminist therapy integrates feminist principles into therapeutic interventions and attributes psychological anguish to sociopolitical and cultural contexts instead of women's flaws (Enns, 2012; Evans & Miller, 2015). Two tenets of feminist therapy that provide a framework for contextualizing the experiences of BCS – the personal is political and honoring women's voices Corey (2017) – will be used to illustrate their applicability.

The personal is political

At the core of feminist therapy is the principle that the personal is political (Enns, 2012). It means that women's psychological issues are embedded in the lived values of a patriarchal and gendered society that disempowers and marginalizes them in political, social, cultural, and economic contexts (Enns, 2012; Evans et al., 2010; Evans & Miller, 2015). These contexts are fraught with difficulties surrounding gender roles and expectations, minority status, power differentials, and socialization experiences. Ultimately, the pressures emanating from these experiences manifest themselves into psychological challenges that women continuously confront. Feminist therapy explores how systems of privilege and power block women from achieving their potential and empowers women to make changes in their lives that promote gender equality (Evans et al., 2010; Pusateri & Headley, 2015). The personal is the political manifests in the lives of BCS in several ways.

Women as sex objects
In Western culture, men shape standards for gender role expectations and female attractiveness. Consequently, a woman's appearance is given continuous agency both by men and by women (Boquiren et al., 2013; Corey, 2017; Evans et al., 2010). Women judge themselves and equate their self-worth with unrealistic standards of beauty, while the weight loss, cosmetic and clothing industries continue to profit handsomely from selling "attractiveness" to them. Society has created different rules for men and women around attractiveness, sexuality, and gender roles and expectations. The societal message is that sex

and sensuality sell. For BCS who are heavily invested in their appearance, yet do not meet the societal standards of beauty, body image, sexuality, body shame and stigma, and body betrayal are pertinent concerns for them (Trachtenberg, 2012).

Women and imperfect bodies
Societal objectification of the breasts is prevalent. Some BCS have lost both breasts. Because society equates a woman's breasts with her sexuality and womanhood, BCS feel devalued because their bodies are "imperfect" as defined by society (Boquiren et al., 2013). BCS struggle with nursing a child, wearing specific styles of clothing, being afraid to look at the surgical body scars, conflicts about how others perceive their missing breasts, treatment from others, and feeling less than womanly. Further, if the BCS decides against breast reconstructive surgery, they are strongly encouraged to reconsider by loved ones and the medical establishment who regard breast reconstruction as a means of preserving survivors' appearance and restoring normalcy (Rubin & Tanenbaum, 2011; Szumacher, 2006). Younger BCS opt for reconstructive surgery for this reason (Campbell-Enns & Woodgate, 2017). Residual effects of chemotherapy and radiation such as hair loss, skin color changes, and weight fluctuations, also cause significant distress (Lewis-Smith et al., 2018; Przezdziecki et al., 2013). BCS self-esteem and culturally ingrained messages about attractiveness shape their reactions to their altered bodies.

Women as child-bearers
The personal is the political resonates with the deeply imbedded cultural imperative that women are created to bear children (Boquiren et al., 2013). For example, women who have not borne children are frequently questioned about such plans. Even more pronounced are negative societal attitudes about women who choose not to have children. Breast loss, sexual dysfunction, and the inability to bear children represent threats to a woman's femininity and reproductive capability (Boquiren et al., 2013). For BCS of childbearing age, these attitudes impact already existing partnered relationships and prospective future relationships, especially if having children is desired (Avis et al., 2005; Howard-Anderson et al., 2012). Embedded in women's cultural socialization is the notion that fertility and childbearing define their person. Infertility threatens their integrity and sense of self. For BCS, this imperative becomes yet another source of distress and an example of the personal being political.

Breast reconstruction
While breast reconstruction is an elective procedure, many BCS feel pressured by their provider to justify their decision against reconstructive breast surgery (Rubin & Tanenbaum, 2011). Physicians must be careful not to suggest that the woman's physical presentation, specifically her breasts, signal wholeness,

physical attractiveness, and femininity. Such action reinforces the dominant culture's perspective and a paternalistic viewpoint. Feminist perspectives call for empowered decision-making and encourage BCS to make their own choices regarding femininity and sexuality (Sulik & Zierkiewicz, 2014). Breast reconstruction is confusing for BCS. Those who decide against it are viewed as de-sexualized; those who chose it, endorse societal norms of attractiveness.

Women's voices are valued and honored

Feminist therapy focuses on honoring the experiences and perspectives of all women, especially those rendered voiceless by marginalization, oppression, and all types of devaluation (Corey, 2017; Enns, 2012). When women are validated, included, speak their truths, make their own choices, and trust their intuition, the gender dialogue shifts to inclusivity and belonging (Evans et al., 2010; Evans & Miller, 2015). The personal becomes political when systemic mechanisms set in place by society continue to give little value to all women's voices. For some BCS, being rendered voiceless is manifested in continued breast cancer treatment disparities, including limited inclusion in cancer trials and research studies, poorer treatment outcomes, and lower breast cancer survival rates.

Limited demographic diversity

Breast cancer studies usually involve White, young, middle-class women who possess the necessary time and participation resources while women from diverse ethnic and socio-economic backgrounds (e.g., older age, women of color, lesbian women, lower socio-economic status, international women) are not frequently included in research protocols and cancer trials (Ashing-Giwa et al., 2004; Meads & Moore, 2013; Rubin & Tanenbaum, 2011; Szumacher, 2006). With data lacking, information on best cancer treatment choices do not include the voices of all women, but just a selected few.

Treatment disparities and survival rates

Black women have higher rates of advanced, aggressive cancer when the cancer is first discovered and higher mortality rates than White women, with a death rate of 42% (DeSantis et al., 2016; Richardson et al., 2016). Breast cancer is the most common cancer and the leading cause of cancer death among Latina women (Rey-Vargas et al., 2019). Black and Latina women are less likely than White women to be screened for breast cancer, are diagnosed later, and are less likely to receive recommended treatments. Asian/Pacific Islanders and White women are screened for cancer at comparable rates (Chen & Li, 2015). Lesbian women are at a higher risk of developing breast cancer because of reproductive and lifestyle risk factors (Meads &

Moore, 2013; Quinn et al., 2015). Further, women 65 and older are less likely to be screened for breast cancer than younger women (Chen & Li, 2015).

Reasons for these health disparities include poverty, communication and language barriers, lack of a primary care provider, lifestyle behavior choices, lack of understanding about healthcare risks, and cultural practices and beliefs (Yedjou et al., 2017). These treatment disparities have impacted the survival rates of women of color and lesbian BCS and represent a serious social justice issue because these women still remain voiceless.

Lack of autonomy and participation in treatment

Shared decision-making represents the gold standard of patient care, where BCS and their medical providers are intimately involved in treatment protocols and outcomes (Rubin & Tanenbaum, 2011; Szumacher, 2006). For some BCS, such participation presents a variety of challenges. Roadblocks such as social class and cultural difficulties, sexual orientation, communication and language challenges, misunderstanding about healthcare risks and cultural practices, provider insensitivity, systemic insensitivity, negative contact with providers, and paternalistic providers, compromise quality care (Ashing-Giwa et al., 2004; Sulik & Zierkiewicz, 2014; Szumacher, 2006). These factors reinforce BCS invisibility in marginalized populations.

Treatment disparities exist among specific communities of BCS and encompass layers of social, psychological, cultural/ethnic, and economic variables. Culturally appropriate, relevant health care must be a right for all BCS and must address the biopsychosocial and cultural barriers outlined that prevent these women from accessing proper care. Listening to and honoring the voices of BCS are powerful treatment tools for accessing their journeys, planning treatment needs, and increasing their survival rates.

Clinical interventions for breast cancer survivors utilizing feminist therapy principles

Gender role analysis

Gender role analysis invites women to explore gender socialization practices on their identities, personhood, and power, including direct and indirect messages focused on "appropriate" gender behaviors, values, and expectations (Corey, 2017; Enns, 2012; Evans & Miller, 2015). Therapists encourage BCS to identify positive and negative messages they receive about beauty, body image, sexuality, and gender role expectations from family, society, and the environment. The information will inform BCS experiences with breast cancer by illustrating how socialization practices have influenced their breast cancer survivorship. Therapists consider asking questions such as: "How did you learn about gender?" "What did you learn about gender?" "In what ways does this information help you to understand your breast cancer experiences?" This dialogue will open up more in-depth exploration to include additional queries on beauty and attractiveness, body image, and sexuality.

Therapists and BCS jointly explore the meanings of health and illness and definitions of attractiveness from a cultural and individual perspective to help BCS distinguish between their own beliefs and those of society (Trachtenberg, 2012). Exploring BCS lived experiences of these meanings gives voice to their truths conceptualized through the lenses of their journey instead of society's narrative.

Reinforcing existing power imbalances and gender role expectations lead to faulty thinking. To address this, therapists and BCS collaborate to identify situations that challenged the BCS core beliefs about gender and role intersectionality. Therapists can teach BCS through empowerment skills, how to change those situations and make new choices. Most importantly, therapists can help BCS understand that even though their experiences were influenced by a society where gender role expectations are ingrained and sometimes difficult to change, BCS have the power to rewrite their individual stories. They are not stuck and can redefine themselves by creating an "after breast cancer" identity that currently defines them.

Gender role intervention

Gender role intervention emphasizes ways that societal gender expectations exacerbate and reinforce distress (Corey, 2017; Enns, 2012; Evans & Miller, 2015). For BCS, distress results from a variety of factors, including the inability to bear children, not conforming to cultural standards of beauty or role strain caused by the debilitating effects of breast cancer (Campbell-Enns & Woodgate, 2017; Howard-Anderson et al., 2012). BCS hear these messages directly, indirectly, and continuously that stepping out of their prescribed roles is not acceptable.

BCS blame themselves for their difficulties instead of looking at external factors. Therapists assist BCS in understanding that their psychological pain is environmentally constructed. When therapists couch distress as caused externally by unjust systems instead of internal flaws, BCS feel less self-blame for their intrapsychic difficulties. Therapists also explain to BCS that they believed these messages because of powerlessness, lack of resources, lack of a voice, societal dictates, or conditioning. By contextualizing BCS experiences in this manner, therapists encourage them to create new messages that are more positive, realistic, empowering, and honest.

Power analysis

Power analysis allows BCS to understand how gendered power differentials limit women's well-being, self-development, choices, and potential (Enns,

2012; Pusateri & Headley, 2015). These power imbalances manifest in a variety of ways including body image concerns, stereotypical gender roles, discrimination, minimal resources, demographic disparities (e.g., race, sexual minority status, age, class, socio-economic status, culture), whether or not to have reconstructive surgery, making treatment decisions, and selecting a provider (Campbell-Enns & Woodgate, 2017; Fingeret et al., 2014; Howard-Anderson et al., 2012; Rubin & Tanenbaum, 2011; Szumacher, 2006). Therapists support the BCS in identifying power they already have but are not aware, and dialogue about how that power can be used to challenge oppressive systems that impact BCS. For example, conversations about decision-making, goal setting, identifying their existing power despite the diagnosis, empowering and supporting their choices to change insensitive providers, refusing reconstructive surgery, and refusing to wear a wig, are compelling. Helping BCS to celebrate their lived experiences and accept their identities as survivors within the context of their own instead of society's expectations, are ways to regain power and create change.

Consciousness raising

Consciousness raising, a principle of feminist therapy, provides a venue for women to create awareness of their experiences with gender-based discrimination, oppression, devaluation, and marginalization (Enns, 2012; Evans & Miller, 2015). It allows women to distinguish between socially dictated and health behavioral choices and to make choices consistent with their needs and desires (Evans et al., 2010; Evans & Miller, 2015). Consciousness raising allows women to share their truths. Consciousness raising groups provide support, camaraderie, commonality of experiences, and linkages to mechanisms for changing oppressive social structures (Corey, 2017; Enns, 2012). Therapists discuss with BCS the benefits of joining such a group. Particularly for BCS who feel voiceless, these groups allow universality of experiences with other survivors, automatic network support, decreased isolation, and opportunities for catharsis (Corey, 2017; Enns, 2012). In addition to consciousness raising groups, therapists refer BCS to specialized groups and organizations that provide support for cancer survivors or to long-term therapy. Diverse women's voices at the center of therapy offer a variety of perspectives, experiences, and truths.

Reframing and relabeling

Feminist therapists view clinical diagnosis as an artifact of patriarchy and conceptualize mental health concerns as the result of intrapsychic issues resulting from socially and culturally imposed systems (Enns, 2012; Evans & Miller, 2015). Therapists reframe psychological distress as a reaction to coping in a stressful, socio-political, and hostile environment, and a conditioned response to oppressive factors (Enns, 2012). Reframing and relabeling moves from blaming the woman to examining social systems and elements in the environment that are responsible (Enns, 2012; Evans & Miller, 2015). For example, if a survivor is experiencing depression and negative body image concerns from breast cancer surgery, the therapist reframes the problem by saying that her angst is a result of society's focus on ideal standards of beauty defined by men, and not an intrapsychic deficiency. Similarly, relabeling retitles the behavior – the BCS repeats to herself that she is courageous for having undergone breast cancer surgery, or she is strong for choosing not to have reconstructive breast surgery. Therapists reinforce and relabel behaviors so that BCS do not internalize unfair societal imperatives.

Commitment to social change

Feminist therapists aim for social change (Corey, 2017; Enns, 2012; Evans & Miller, 2015). Therapists discuss with BCS how their identities (race, gender, sexual orientation, religion) have caused oppressive suffering intersecting with their experiences with breast cancer. As members of a marginalized group, BCS join with others to address similar concerns. Advocacy is critical to feminist therapy because personal freedom cannot occur without social change (Enns, 2012; Evans & Miller, 2015). Therapists help BCS to identify their individual advocacy interests and initiatives and use their extensive knowledge to direct BCS to a variety of resources. Some advocacy platforms include volunteering, lobbying activities, community breast cancer education, conference presentations on surviving breast cancer, and conducting and presenting breast cancer research.

Empowerment through photovoice

Photovoice empowers BCS to shape their personal breast cancer narrative through the use of photographs (Liebenberg, 2018; Wang & Burris, 1994). Photovoice is done through recording images that depict common problems, evaluating dialogue around the issues, and using the information to implement change. Photovoice is used to explore many facets of breast cancer and body image. For example, the photographs capture snapshots that are meaningful to survivors, such as their hair growing back in stages, chemotherapy treatments, and pictures of their scars. Discussing the pictures as part of therapy enhances BCS's ability to express their needs and emotions and gives voice to their voice. This technique allows therapists to contextualize BCS feelings better and strengthen the therapeutic support by negotiating the challenges of breast cancer and body image (Sloan et al., 2018). Photovoice promotes the precepts of feminist theory as it provides a vehicle to recognize, analyze, and challenge oppressive systems that influence breast cancer treatment and body image (Mayfield-Johnson et al., 2014).

Self-advocacy and treatment navigation

Individualized psychoeducation and negotiating the healthcare system are paramount when seeking to empower and inform BCS (Freeman & Rodriguez, 2011). Therapists are encouraged to coordinate care with the oncologist and other medical providers. The process will support the continuity of care received by BCS, allow therapists to assist BCS in understanding the role of the medical team, empower survivors to self-advocate any treatment concerns, and reframe the pathology-oriented processes of the medical model of care (Szumacher, 2006). Treatment navigation is used by multidisciplinary medical teams to guide patient care, eliminate barriers to resources, and encourage expedient diagnosis and treatment through a public intervention service. Treatment navigation with the therapist helps BCS avoid barriers related to access, quality of care, communication, financial limitations, and mistrust of the medical community (Freeman & Rodriguez, 2011). It is important that therapists understand strategies that support successful treatment navigation and convey them to BCS. For example, therapists can teach BCS assertiveness skills that facilitate self-guided healthcare and personal advocacy.

Helping medical providers understand the sociopolitical contexts of breast cancer

The multidisciplinary treatment team approach brings together varying disciplines to provide comprehensive medical care to BCS. The treatment team approach demonstrates an orientation similar to that of feminist theory. Both encourage a multidisciplinary strength-focused approach, value diverse perspectives, and are focused on creating egalitarian relationships (Shao et al., 2019). Therapists can help the team to identify the parallel goals that exist between feminist theory and the treatment team model of patient care. Understanding these similarities can help the team more readily identify and contextualize existing sociopolitical aspects of treatment in both a broad and specific patient context. In a broad context, therapists support the treatment team in understanding how social constructs, including race and gender, dictate which disorders are researched, what treatment is available, and where access to treatment is provided (Rogers & Kelly, 2011). In a specific context, therapists outline the survivor's individualized needs with respect to the distribution of power in the patient-physician relationship, traditional perceptions of gender roles, as well as socio-economic status and other disenfranchising systems that impact the treatment process (Sulik & Zierkiewicz, 2014).

Further, when participating with the treatment team, therapists can suggest the implementation of several strategies that promote increased survivorship. Kline et al. (2018) outlined recommendations to support BCS that include integrative psychological care, accessible and cost-effective primary and palliative services, and the development and education of staff that promote person-centered coordinated care. Incorporating feminist theory into treatment planning and decision-making models for BCS gives therapists the opportunity to share resources and education on a variety of issues while improving the overall quality of care BCS receive. Therapists can provide information regarding constructs of power and patient choice. In this forum, therapists can also challenge normative ideas about family, gender, and other sociopolitical concerns that arise (Szumacher, 2006).

Implications for practice

BCS experience life-altering body image and biopsychosocial changes that come with a diagnosis of breast cancer. There are several implications for practitioners beyond the interventions described previously. First, improved continuity of care and integrative treatment planning that addresses not only the medical but also the body image, biopsychosocial, and cultural needs of BCS must become the standard of care. If not, then adequate treatment will continue to be reserved for a select few survivors. Additionally, cultural competency training to ensure appropriate clinical care and understanding of factors responsible for the high mortality rates among underrepresented BCS is essential. Finally, practitioners are called to lend their voices to collaborative grassroots efforts, community campaigns, public health initiatives, and educational partnerships that address the needs of marginalized BCS. This will help to improve BCS quality of life and survival rates.

Limitations and future research

There are several limitations to this manuscript. First, the information is not generalizable to all breast cancer survivors (e.g., men, older women, ethnically and sexually diverse women, women of lower SES). Another major limitation is that much of the extant literature on BCS, including data in this manuscript, focused on young Caucasian BCS and lacks a balanced, diverse perspective (Ashing-Giwa et al., 2004; Fingeret et al., 2013; Paterson et al., 2016); therefore, its applicability to women of diverse demographics is limited. Research continues to outline the disparities in breast cancer and risk factor rates, especially among racial and ethnic minority women. Increased research is necessary to understand the causes of the disparities and how to reduce them so that all women have access to culturally appropriate and effective breast cancer treatment. Additionally, BCS lived experiences can be very dissimilar across identities, and body image may not be an integral concern as highlighted. Finally, this was not an empirical study; therefore, research focusing on BCS utilizing empirically sound methodology, addressing treatment and body image disparities, and focusing on culturally relevant treatment protocols and interventions for BCS is vital. Research through the feminist lens honoring the experiences and voices of a broad spectrum of BCS provides practitioners with a better understanding of the challenges and additional factors to consider for treatment and survivorship.

Conclusion

A breast cancer diagnosis carries medical and biopsychosocial challenges that encompass more than body image concerns. Despite existing research, specific populations of BCS remain underserved, as evidenced by their increased mortality rates and limited inclusion in research. Gaps in research, funding, and educational initiatives still exist. Thus, practitioners who work with BCS are responsible for providing competent, quality, culturally sensitive clinical and therapeutic care, while exploring a variety of initiatives designed to increase BCS life satisfaction and survival rates. Addressing these gaps is not only a feminist therapy imperative but also a social justice responsibility.

ORCID

Levette S Scott http://orcid.org/0000-0002-7714-7102
Raheem J. Paxton http://orcid.org/0000-0001-9430-7051

References

Archangelo, S., Sabino, N., Veiga, D., Garcia, E., & Ferreira, L. (2019). Sexuality, depression, and body image after breast reconstruction. *Clinics (Sao Paulo, Brazil)*, 74, e883–e888. https://doi.org/10.6061/clinics/2019/e883

Ashing, K. T., George, M., & Jones, V. (2018). Health-related quality of life and care satisfaction outcomes: Informing psychosocial oncology care among Latina and African- American young breast cancer survivors. *Psycho-Oncology*, 27(4), 1213–1220. https://doi.org/10.1002/pon.4650

Ashing-Giwa, K. T., Padilla, G., Tejero, J., Kraemer, J., Wright, K., Coscarelli, A., Clayton, S., Williams, I., & Hills, D. (2004). Understanding the breast cancer experience of women: A qualitative study of African American, Asian American, Latina, and White cancer survivors. *Psycho-Oncology*, 13(6), 408–428. https://doi.org/10.1002/pon.750

Avis, N., Crawford, S., & Manuel, J. (2005). Quality of life among younger women with breast cancer. *Journal of Clinical Oncology*, 15(15), 3322–3330. https://doi.org/10.1200/JCO.2005.05.130

Bazzi, A. R., Whorms, D. S., King, D. S., & Potter, J. (2015). Adherence to mammography screening guidelines among transgender persons and sexual minority women. *American Journal of Public Health, 105*(11), 2356–2358. https://doi.org/10.2105/AJPH.2015.302851

Boehmer, U., Glickman, M., Winter, M., & Clark, M. A. (2013). Lesbian and bisexual women's adjustment after a breast cancer diagnosis. *Journal of the American Psychiatric Nurses Association, 19*(5), 280–292. https://doi.org/10.1177/1078390313504587

Boing, L., Pereira, G. S., Araújo, C., Sperandio, F. F., Loch, M., Bergmann, A., Guimarães, A., & Guimarães, A. C. D. A. (2019). Factors associated with depression symptoms in women after breast cancer. *Revista De Saúde Pública, 53*(30), 1–12. https://doi.org/10.11606/s1518-8787.2019053000786

Boquiren, V. M., Esplen, M. J., Wong, J., Toner, B., & Warner, E. (2013). Exploring the influence of gender-role socialization and objectified body consciousness on body image disturbance in breast cancer survivors. *Psycho-Oncology, 22*(10), 2177–2185. https://doi.org/10.1002/pon.3271

Campbell-Enns, H. J., & Woodgate, R. L. (2017). The psychosocial experiences of women with breast cancer across the lifespan: A systematic review. *Psycho-Oncology, 26*(11), 1711–1721. https://doi.org/10.1002/pon.4281

Cancer facts & figures (2019). American Cancer Society. https://www.cancer.org/content/dam/cancer-org/research/cancer-facts-and-statistics/annual-cancer-facts-and-figures/2019/cancer-facts-and-figures-2019.pdf

Cash, T. F. (2011). Cognitive-behavioral perspectives on body image. In *Body image: A handbook of science, practice, and prevention* (2nd ed., pp. 39–47). Guilford Press.

Center for Disease Control and Prevention. (2016). *Female rate of cancer deaths by race/ethnicity*. The United States Cancer Statistics. https://gis.cdc.gov/Cancer/USCS/DataViz.html

Chen, L., & Li, C. (2015). Racial disparities in breast cancer diagnosis and treatment by hormone receptor and HER2 status. *Cancer Epidemiology and Prevention Biomarkers, 24*(11), 1666–1672. https://doi.org/10.1158/1055-9965.EPI-15-0293

Corey, G. (2017). Feminist therapy. In *Theory and practice of counseling and psychotherapy* (9th ed., pp. 343–354). Cengage Learning.

Dean, L. T., Moss, S. L., Rollinson, S. I., Jaramillo, L. F., Paxton, R. J., & Owczarzak, J. T. (2019). Patient recommendations for reducing long-lasting economic burden after breast cancer. *Cancer, 125*(11), 1929–1940. https://doi.org/10.1002/cncr.32012

DeSantis, C., Fedewa, S., Sauer, A., Kramer, J., Smith, R., & Jemal, A. (2016). Breast cancer statistics, 2015: Convergence of incidence rates between Black and White women. *CA: A Cancer Journal for Clinicians, 66*(1), 31–42. https://doi.org/10.3322/caac.21320

Enns, C. Z & Williams, E.N. (2012). Feminist approaches to counseling. In *The Oxford handbook of counseling psychology* (pp. 434–459). Oxford University Press.

Evans, K., & Miller, M. (2015). Feminist therapy. In I. Marini & M. Stebnicki (Eds.), *The professional counselor's desk reference* (2nd ed., pp. 247–251). Springer Publishing.

Evans, K., Kincade, E., & Seem, S. (2010). *Introduction to feminist therapy: Strategies for social and individual change* (pp. 2–22). Sage Publishing.

Fingeret, M. C., Nipomnick, S. W., Crosby, M. A., & Reece, G. P. (2013). Developing a theoretical framework to illustrate associations among patient satisfaction, body image, and quality of life for women undergoing breast reconstruction. *Cancer Treatment Reviews, 39*(6), 673–681. https://doi.org/10.1016/j.ctrv.2012.12.010

Fingeret, M. C., Teo, I., & Epner, D. E. (2014). Managing body image difficulties of adult cancer patients: Lessons from available research. *Cancer, 120*(5), 633–641. https://doi.org/10.1002/cncr.28469

Fobair, P., & Spiegel, D. (2009). Concerns about sexuality after breast cancer. *Cancer Journal, 15*(1), 19–26. https://doi.org/10.1097/PPO.0b013e31819587bb

Fobair, P., Stewart, S. L., Chang, S., D'Onofrio, C., Banks, P. J., & Bloom, J. R. (2006). Body image and sexual problems in young women with breast cancer. *Psycho- Oncology, 15*(7), 579–594. https://doi.org/10.1002/pon.991

Foy, K., Fisher, J., Lustberg, M., Gray, D., DeGraffinreid, C., & Paskett, E. (2018). Disparities in breast cancer tumor characteristics, treatment, time to treatment, and survival probability among African American and White women. *NPJ Breast Cancer, 4*(1), 1–6. https://doi.org/10.1038/s41523-018-0059-5

Freeman, H., & Rodriguez, R. (2011). History and principles of patient navigation. *Cancer, 117*(S15), 3537–3540. https://doi.org/10.1002/cncr.26262

Grecucci, A., Pappaianni, E., Siugzdaite, R., Theuninck, A., Frederick, J., & Job, R. (2015). Mindful emotion regulation: Exploring the neurocognitive mechanisms behind mindfulness. *BioMed - Research International, 2015,* 670724. https//doi.101155./2015/670724.

Howard-Anderson, J., Ganz, P. A., Bower, J. E., & Stanton, A. L. (2012). Quality of life, fertility concerns, and behavioral health outcomes in younger breast cancer survivors: A systematic review. *Journal of the National Cancer Institute, 104*(5), 386–405. https://doi.org/10.1093/jnci/djr541

Inhestern, L., & Bergelt, C. (2018). When a mother has cancer: Strains and resources of affected families from the mother's and father's perspective - A qualitative study. *BMC Women's Health, 18*(1), 1–11. https://doi.org/10.1186/s12905-018-0562-8

Jing, L., Zhang, C., Li, W., Jin, F., & Wang, A. (2019). Incidence and severity of sexual dysfunction among women with breast cancer: A meta-analysis based on female sexual function index. *Supportive Care in Cancer, 27*(4), 1171–1180. https://doi.org/10.1007/s00520-019-04667-7

King, R. K., Alexander, R. G., Tan-Gregory, A., Donahue, E. J., Kimbrough-Sugick,,, Betancourt, J. R., & KIMBROUGH-SUGICK, J. (2008). A plan for action: Key perspectives from the racial/ethnic disparities strategy forum. *Milbank Quarterly, 86*(2), 241–272. https://doi.org/10.1111/j.1468-0009.2008.00521.x

Kline, R. M., Arora, N. K., Bradley, C. J., Brauer, E. R., Graves, D. L., Lunsford, N. B., McCabe, M., Nasso, S., Nekhlyudov, L., Rowland, J., Schear, R., & Ganz, P. (2018). Long-term survivorship care after cancer treatment-summary of a 2017 national cancer policy forum workshop. *Journal of the National Cancer Institute, 110*(12), 1300–1310. https://doi.org/10.1093/jnci/djy176

Lewis-Smith, H., Diedrichs, P. C., & Harcourt, D. (2018). A pilot study of a body image intervention for breast cancer survivors. *Body Image, 27,* 21–31. https://doi.org/10.1016/j.bodyim.2018.08.006

Liebenberg, L. (2018). Thinking critically about photovoice: Achieving empowerment and social change. *International Journal of Qualitative Methods, 17*(1), 1–9. https://doi.org/10.1177/1609406918757631

Mayfield-Johnson, S., Rachal, J. R., & Butler III, J. (2014). "When we learn better, we do better:" Describing changes in empowerment through photovoice among community health advisors in a breast and cervical cancer health promotion program in Mississippi and Alabama. *Adult Education Quarterly, 64*(2), 91–109. https://doi.org/10.1177/0741713614521862

Meads, C., & Moore, D. (2013). Breast cancer in lesbians and bisexual women: Systematic review of incidence, prevalence, and risk studies. *BMC Public Health, 13*(1), 1–11. https://doi.org/10.1186/1471-2458-13-1127

Moreira, H., & Canavarro, M. C. (2010). A longitudinal study about body image and psychosocial adjustment of breast cancer patients during the course of the disease. *European Journal of Oncology Nursing, 14*(4), 263–270. https://doi.org/10.1016/j.ejon.2010.04.001

Oberguggenberger, A., Martini, C., Huber, N., Fallow, L., Hubalek, M., Daniaux, M., Meraner, V., Holzner, B., Sztankay, M., Gamper, E., & Meraner, V. (2017). Self-reported sexual health: Breast cancer survivors compared to women from the general population – An observational study. *BMC Cancer, 17*(1), 1–9. https://doi.org/10.1186/s12885-017-3580-2

Patel-Kerai, G., Harcourt, D., Rumsey, N., Naqvi, H., & White, P. (2017). The psychosocial experiences of breast cancer amongst Black, South Asian, and White survivors: Do differences exist between ethnic groups? *Psycho-Oncology, 26*(4), 515–522. https://doi.org/10.1002/pon.4187

Paterson, C. L., Lengacher, C. A., Donovan, K. A., Kip, K. E., & Tofthagen, C. S. (2016). Body image in younger breast cancer survivors: A systematic review. *Cancer Nursing, 39*(E39–), E58. https://doi.org/10.1186/s12885-017-3580-2

Pikler, V., & Winterowd, C. (2003). Racial and Body Image Differences in Coping for Women Diagnosed With Breast Cancer.. *Health Psychology., 22*(6), 632–637. https://doi.org/10.1037/0278-6133.22.6.632

Przezdziecki, A., Sherman, K. A., Baillie, A., Taylor, A., Foley, E., & Stalgis-Balinski, K. (2013). My changed body: Breast cancer, body image, distress, and self-compassion. *Psycho-Oncology, 22*(8), 1872–1879. https://doi.org/10.1002/pon.3230

Pusateri, C., & Headley, C. (2015). Feminist therapy. In E. Neukrug (Ed.), *The sage encyclopedia of theory in counseling and psychotherapy* (pp. 414–419). Sage Publications.

Quinn, G. P., Sanchez, J. A., Sutton, S. K., Vadaparampil, S. T., Nguyen, G. T., Green, B. L., Kanetsky, P. A., & Schabath, M. B. (2015). Cancer and lesbian, gay, bisexual, transgender/transsexual,and queer/questioning (LGBTQ) populations. *CA: A Cancer Journal for Clinicians, 65*(5), 384–400. https://doi.org/10.3322/caac.21288

Rey-Vargas, L., Sanabria-Salas, C., Fejerman, L., & Serrano-Gómez, S. (2019). Risk factors for triple-negative breast cancer among Latina women. *Cancer Epidemiology and Prevention Biomarkers, 28*(11), 1771–1783. https://doi.org/10.1158/1055-9965.EPI-19-0035

Rezaei, M., Elyasi, F., Janbabai, G., Moosazadeh, M., & Hamzehgardeshi, Z. (2016). Factors influencing body image in women with breast cancer: A comprehensive literature review. *Iranian Red Crescent Medical Journal, 18*(10), 1–28. https://doi.org/10.5812/ircmj.39465

Richardson, L., Henley, J., Miller, J., Massetti, G., & Thomas, C. (2016). Patterns and trends in Black-White differences in breast cancer incidence and mortality - United States, 1999 – 2013. *MMWR, 65*(40), 1093–1098. https://doi.org/10.15585/mmwr.mm6540a1

Rogers, J., & Kelly, U. A. (2011). Feminist intersectionality: Bringing social justice to health disparities research. *Nursing Ethics, 18*(3), 397–407. https://doi.org/10.1177/0969733011398094

Rotter, J., Spencer, J. C., & Wheeler, S. B. (2018). Financial toxicity in advanced and metastatic cancer: Overburdened and underprepared. *Journal of Oncology Practice, 15*(4), 300–307. https://doi.org/10.1200/JOP.18.00518

Rubin, L. R., & Tanenbaum, M. (2011). "Does that make me a woman?": Breast cancer, mastectomy, and breast reconstruction decisions among sexual minority women. *Psychology of Women Quarterly, 35*(3), 401–414. https://doi.org/10.1177/0361684310395606

Shao, J., Rodrigues, M., Corter, A. L., & Baxter, N. N. (2019). Multidisciplinary care of breast cancer patients: A scoping review of multidisciplinary styles, processes, and outcomes. *Current Oncology, 26*(3), 385–397. https://doi.org/10.3747/co.26.4713

Sloan, S., Teti, M., & Benson, J. (2018). Redefining body image after breast cancer: A photovoice study. *Innovation in Aging, 2*(suppl_1), 275–276. https://doi.org/10.1093/geroni/igy023.1019

Sulik, G., & Zierkiewicz, E. (2014). Gender, power, and feminisms in breast cancer advocacy: Lessons from the United States and Poland. *Journal of Gender and Power*, *1*(1), 111–145.

Szumacher, E. (2006). The feminist approach in the decision-making process for treatment of women with breast cancer. *Annals-Academy of Medicine Singapore*, *9*(35), 655–661.

Trachtenberg, L. (2012). Identity reformulation among young women with breast cancer (Order No. MR92952). Available from ProQuest Dissertations & Theses Global. (1328168540). http://nclive.org.ezproxy.nccu.edu/cgi-bin/nclsm?url=http://search.proquest.com.ezproxy.nccu.edu/dissertations-theses/identity-reformulation-among-young-women-with/docview/1328168540/se-2?accountid=12713

Van Puymbroeck, M., Schmid, A., Shinew, K. J., & Hsieh, P. C. (2011). Influence of hatha yoga on physical activity constraints, physical fitness, and body image of breast cancer survivors: A pilot study. *International Journal of Yoga Therapy*, *21*(1), 49–60. https://doi.org/10.17761/ijyt.21.1.n852143rv21x188u

Wang, C., & Burris, M. A. (1994). Empowerment through photo novella: Portraits of participation. *Health Education Quarterly*, *21*(2), 171–186. https://doi.org/10.1177/109019819402100204

White, C. A. (2002). Body images in oncology. In C. Baker & E. Wertheim (Eds..), *Body image: A handbook of theory, research, and clinical practice* (pp. 379–386). The Guilford Press. https://10.1080/1064026039021873

Yedjou, C., Tchounwou, B., Payton, M., Miele, L., Fonseca, D., Lowe, L., & Alo, R. (2017). Assessing the racial and ethnic disparities in breast cancer mortality in the United States. *International Journal of Environmental Research and Public Health*, *14*(5), 486–498. https://doi.org/10.3390/ijerph14050486

Gender Roles and the Family Life Cycle: The Case of Women with Cancer

Larra Petersen, Theresa Kruczek and Angela Shaffner

SUMMARY
A woman's diagnosis of cancer affects the family system by requiring families to accommodate new daily routines, redistribute roles, develop a new sense of normalcy, and anticipate future changes in family functioning. Gender-role socialization influences the family's ability to adapt to the myriad of changes necessary during the woman's treatment and recovery from cancer. This article integrates knowledge of gender-role socialization within the context of family systems principles and family life cycle stages in order to provide a framework for working with female cancer patients and their families. A case application exemplifying the unique struggle of women diagnosed within the context of the family life cycle is provided.

Women have a one in three lifetime risk of developing cancer (Kayser, Sormanti, & Strainchamps, 1999). Lung, breast, and colorectal cancers account for the highest cancer death rates among women in North America (American Cancer Society, 2003). It is estimated that in 2003 over 211,000 new cases of breast cancer alone will be diagnosed in women (American Cancer Society, 2003). The clinical course of cancer is unique from other illnesses, and influences the situational stressors patients face (Nicholas & Veach, 2000). The disease process begins like other illnesses with initial symptoms, followed by a medical workup and diagnosis. Treatment decisions are then based on the stage of the cancer and can be especially difficult when the disease is in an advanced stage. Unlike many other diseases, often there is not one clearly best treatment option. Women must consider their unique personal, situational, and life stage variables within the context of quality of life versus quantity of life. Treatment may last weeks or months and the side effects from treatment can be debilitating. When treatment has been "effective" the cancer patient undergoes a period of rehabilitation and remission. In these cases, women may experience cancer as a chronic illness, with long-term disabilities. For others, recurrence and further treatment will occur, and this cycle may repeat several times. If the disease continues to progress, the focus shifts to palliative care and quality rather than quantity of life (Nicholas & Veach, 2000).

Cancer patients in general struggle with issues of remission, relapse, deterioration, long-term survival and fear/uncertainty about recurrence (Lederberg, 1998). Female cancer patients not only have to deal with the general issues related to cancer, but also gender-specific issues. Women must make treatment decisions that affect their body image (e.g., lumpectomy vs. mastectomy) and future reproductive options. Women in remission may also struggle with quality of life issues specifically related to their cancer treatment such as lymphedema, following breast cancer surgery (Radina & Armer, 2001). While women with cancer face the aforementioned challenges, they also encounter a myriad of social and environmental influences on their adaptation to the illness. Few studies have investigated the effect of a woman's cancer within the context of one of the most significant sources of social influence, her family. The literature that is available highlights the reciprocal nature of the effect of cancer on the overall functioning of the woman and her family.

The diagnosis of cancer requires significant adaptability for a woman because she must carry on family and life responsibilities while also attending to her own illness. Likewise, cancer limits a woman's personal and interpersonal functioning in ways that require the family system to accommodate new daily routines, redistribute roles, develop a new sense of normalcy, offer her emotional support and anticipate future changes in family functioning (Lewis & Hammond, 1992). The family's ability to adapt to these changes significantly affects her treatment and recovery process. The woman with cancer can focus more on self-care when her family provides her with greater instrumental and emotional support (Jacobs et al., 1998; Veach, Nicholas, & Barton, 2002). The following case example is provided to illustrate the reciprocal nature of the effect of cancer on one woman and her family.

Case study

"Patricia" is a 42-year-old, divorced, Caucasian female diagnosed with stage IV breast cancer. During her initial diagnosis, she had surgery to remove a large tumor. Following this surgery, "things got back to normal" for a while and she returned to work. However, a few months later she began experiencing soreness in her back which led to the identification of her recurrence of cancer. She reported feeling shocked and stressed, and she felt the recurrence was more difficult to cope with than the initial diagnosis. Patricia faced many disconcerting questions. First and foremost, she questioned who would care for her 11-year-old son, Jason, while she had her radiation treatments. During Patricia's initial diagnosis and treatment, her ex-mother-in-law helped with his care. However, her former mother-in-law's recent diagnosis with colon cancer prevented her from currently providing significant support. Furthermore, Patricia divorced her first husband, Jason's father, ten years previously when Jason was an infant. Jason rarely saw his father, even though they lived in the same community. Patricia attributed this lack of contact to the father's girlfriend's jealous feelings and lack of commitment to Jason's care. However, Patricia was engaged to Charles, who had a good relationship with Jason. Jason referred to Charles as "Dad" and indicated that he enjoyed their time together. Patricia and Charles planned on marrying in the near future, although the date was tentative due to uncertainty about her course of treatment. Patricia described Charles as supportive of her and her struggles with cancer. In addition to the support from Charles, Patricia's mother also provided some instrumental support, but little emotional support. Specifically, she helped Patricia with cooking and housework. Although Patricia required continued assistance and support, she hoped to return to work soon, since she identified experiencing financial stress and pressure to provide for her family.

Patricia's radiation oncologist referred her to a psychotherapist for evaluation of her psychosocial adjustment to her illness. The counselor met with her son as well, since Patricia was concerned about his adjustment to her illness. Her concerns about him arose after the school counselor called to inform her that Jason was frequently tearful at school. Patricia indicated he never displayed these feelings at home. Through counseling it became clear that Patricia's illness was disruptive to her family and life roles and that she was having difficulty adapting to her illness. In particular, Patricia emphasized her disappointment with the lack of informational support that she received from her medical providers regarding her prognosis and the potential effect of that prognosis on her family plans. As her prognosis was poor, Patricia was forced to consider options for her son after her death. She primarily considered two options for him: living with a maternal aunt and uncle, or moving into his dad's home.

In addition to concerns about her death, she identified that the family structure was shifting as Jason had begun to adopt a caretaking role. Specifically, he had begun making dinner and caring for his mother when she was fatigued and weak. She recognized this occurrence as a breached generational boundary, but in the face of limited resources was uncertain how to decrease the burden on her son. In addition, Jason was struggling with the normative developmental challenges of establishing his identity. For example, as he began adopting communal roles not typically expected from a child his age, he was at risk for confusion about healthy roles in adult-adult relationships. A concern was that this childhood pattern of relating could lead to dependency in his adult intimate relationships.

Treatment involved collaborating with the client and utilizing various strategies for maintaining healthy expression of both focus on self (agency) and others (communion) for all members. Counseling was used to provide a forum for discussion on the agentic and communal needs for Patricia and her family. For instance, Patricia was encouraged to demonstrate agency in seeking out informational support from her medical providers. She also was encouraged to exercise agency in two other areas: making treatment decisions based on her quality and quantity of life concerns and identifying her preference for who would care for Jason after her death.

Through this process Patricia identified that her fiancé, Charles, provided the majority of her emotional support and care for Jason. However, she identified problems with her social network and communion needs. Therefore, she was encouraged to increase communion by expanding her emotional resource base and developing a stronger support network among her friends and spiritual community.

She also used counseling to devise strategies to communicate more frequently and effectively with her ex-husband and extended family in order to meet Jason's needs for relational functioning, given the impending loss of his mother. Ultimately, the intervention strategies were designed to address the effect of gender-role issues on family functioning for Patricia when coping with her cancer.

Gender-role socialization and cancer

This case highlights many of the unique issues faced by women with cancer, particularly the struggle to balance agency and communion. Bakan (1966) postulated two fundamental modalities of human existence related to masculinity and femininity: agency and communion. Agency refers to being independent, active, competitive, decisive, committed (to goals), self-confident, and self-assured. Communion includes being emotional, gentle, helpful, kind, warm, aware (of feelings), and sympathetic (Spence, Helmreich, & Holahan, 1979). Early theorists investigating agency and communion viewed agentic traits as more positive when expressed in males and communal traits more positive when expressed by females (Buss, 1990; Helgeson, 1993; McCreary & Korabic, 1994; Spence et al., 1979). Although current research acknowledges the positive nature of the agency and communion constructs, it also identifies the undesirable or unmitigated components of the traits and the disproportionate effect of these traits on men and women, particularly in the areas of interpersonal relationships and psychological well-being (Helgeson, 1994). Specifically, Spence and colleagues (1979) identify unmitigated agency, which is more common in males, as being the most socially undesirable aspect of agency. Helgeson and Fritz (2000) note that unmitigated agency and agency have the commonality of focus on self but the unmitigated construct includes the focus on the self to the exclusion of others. In contrast, unmitigated communion, which is more commonly identified among women, involves two features of concern in relation to interpersonal functioning: over-involvement and self-neglect (Helgeson, 1994; Fritz & Helgeson, 1998). Consistent with gender-role theory, individuals possessing the unmitigated traits have more difficulty adjusting to cancer (Helgeson & Lepore, 1997; Piro et al., 2001). While gender socialization is not as rigid today as in previous generations, studies show that socialization continues to shape gender-role behaviors (Jacklin, 1989).

Gender-role socialization is the primary process contributing to an imbalance in household responsibilities within couples and families (Freidan, 1997). Traditionally, women have carried a disproportionate burden with regard to household tasks. The imbalance becomes more evident and problematic in the case of cancer. Specifically, the diagnosis of a woman's cancer often requires shifts in family roles with regard to instrumental behaviors, such as household chores and childcare. The family's ability to meet the instrumental and emotional needs of a woman with cancer is, in part, influenced by gender-role socialization. Further, many women try to maintain all pre-cancer tasks and resist asking for help in an attempt to avoid further change and perceived additional stress to the family system (Vess, Moreland, & Schwebel, 1985). Reallocation of role responsibility is easier in family systems demonstrating gender role flexibility. Essentially in healthy families, when the female cancer patient asks for assistance, members respond by redistributing tasks among other capable members, regardless of gender.

Family systems and the family life cycle

The effect of gender-role socialization on the healthy adjustment of women and their families to the diagnosis and treatment of cancer must be understood within the context of family systems theory and the family life cycle. Family systems theory, the application of general systems theory to family functioning, is the dominant model for investigating the effect of stress on the family system (Jacobs et al., 1998). Family systems theory focuses on the extent to which the family system changes its structure and functions across the life cycle in response to both normative developmental changes and stressors, such as cancer (Goldenberg & Goldenberg, 1998; Nichols & Swartz, 1995; Olson & Lavee, 1989). Carter and McGoldrick's (1989) family life cycle theory suggests the female cancer patient is part of a multigenerational system moving vertically (patterns of relating transmitted across generations) and horizontally (normative development and unpredictable stressors) through the life cycle. The interaction of the vertical and horizontal axes occurs when past patterns guide present crisis appraisal, resource management, and expectation of success or failure (Lederberg, 1998). For example, if a grandparent has suffered greatly from complications to cancer treatment, then the woman with cancer and her family are more likely to react strongly to her diagnosis and treatment of cancer because of their past experience and assumptions about the progression of the illness. Therefore, addressing unique family patterns arising in family systems is important for healthy adjustment in families.

Family systems and cancer

Healthy adjustment in families where a woman has cancer depends on the core systems principles of cohesion, adaptability/flexibility, communication, and family roles (Goldenberg & Goldenberg, 1998; Veach et al., 2002), and these principles must be understood within the context of the family lifecycle (Carter & McGoldrick, 1989). First, cohesion refers to the emotional connection family members feel towards one another (Veach et al., 2002). In healthy families, the members remain individuated from but connected to each other. In the case of a woman with cancer, her family would remain involved in her care while continuing obligatory life tasks, such as work or school. In contrast, unhealthy families show patterns where members are enmeshed or disengaged. As Sherman and Simonton (2001) note, it is important to assess and address both enmeshment and disengagement because of their negative effect on cancer adjustment.

Enhancing cohesion in disengaged families with cancer is essential because a cohesive family is better able to adapt to the pressures of the illness by shifting roles, responsibilities, and boundaries over the course of the illness (Sherman & Simonton, 2001). Disengaged family members may show a tendency to move further away from the woman in times of stress or crisis (Sherman & Simonton, 2001). The process of outreach and involvement of the disengaged family members should be gradual. One relatively nonthreatening way to involve a disengaged family member of a woman with cancer is to have them take her to initial medical appointments. This low level of involvement begins building bridges between the family and the disengaged member while paving the way for increased involvement and support as her treatment progresses.

Likewise, enhancing differentiation is important in enmeshed families in order to avoid the family becoming engulfed by efforts to accommodate the illness (Rolland, 1989; Sherman & Simonton, 2001; Veach et al., 2002). The diagnosis and treatment of cancer eclipses all else in the family when the woman becomes the central component of family functioning. Individual members become focused almost exclusively on the emotional and physical needs of the woman with cancer (Sherman & Simonton, 2001). Conversely, the unspoken rules of an enmeshed family can dictate subjugation of the woman's needs in an attempt to maintain all pre-illness routines. When the woman subjugates her cancer treatment needs in order to maintain a pre-illness façade there is a collective denial of the illness. Ultimately, these families should be encouraged to maintain a balanced perspective which highlights non-illness interests, strengths and resources of the female cancer patient as well as other family members while meeting the instrumental and emotional needs of the woman with cancer. Healthy differentiation is particularly important in coping with cancer in order to avoid caregiver burnout and minimize the risk of suppressing the woman's role as a contributing member of the family (Rolland, 1989; Veach et al., 2002).

The family's adaptability in response to the illness is also important for healthy adjustment to a woman's cancer diagnosis and treatment. Jacobs and colleagues (1998) describe a healthy family as cohesive, integrated, and self-stabilizing. Healthy families demonstrate a resilient capacity to change, manifest by learning new ways of solving problems or modifying roles in response to stressors such as cancer. Patterson (1988) proposed the Family Adjustment and Adaptation Response (FAAR) Model to describe healthy adaptation to unexpected stress, such as a diagnosis with cancer. The diagnosis and subsequent treatment causes a crisis until the family develops new resources or coping strategies to deal with the stress of the illness. In particular, reducing the number or stressors addressed by the family and reframing the meaning of the stressors for the family can facilitate healthy adaptation to her cancer.

Typical stressors for women with cancer often involve quality of life issues resulting from undergoing adjuvant therapies (chemotherapy and radiation therapy) and secondary effects from cancer (e.g., lymphedema, or fluid buildup in tissues surrounding removed lymph nodes, typical in breast cancer survivors).

Women coping with cancer also often struggle with balancing their increased dependence on others with the sense of identity they historically have gained from independent responsibility for family matters (Allen & Hawkins, 1999). In particular, family members may foster unhealthy adaptation and unintentionally hinder the woman's functional recovery by encouraging her to remain physically inactive during the adjuvant treatment process (Bolger et al., 1996).

Healthy adaptation for these women and their families will involve making adjustments to the tasks the woman is able to successfully complete, rather than encouraging her to avoid them (Radina & Armer, 2001). For example, when a woman experiences lymphedema, she will not be able to lift more than 10 pounds, make repetitive movements, or have full mobility in the affected arm. Therefore, family members need to be patient with the increased time it takes her to complete tasks or she may need facilitative devices to perform tasks. However, her ability to successfully complete the tasks in a modified fashion not only enhances her sense of agency, but also enables her to remain a valuable resource within the family. In some cases, the woman will need to rely on family members or even outside agencies for assistance with household tasks and treatment. When this happens, healthy adaptation can be facilitated by clear communication about both the logistics of realigned responsibilities and the emotional effect of these changes on all family members (Bolger et al., 1996).

Furthermore, it is important to foster healthy communication in families with cancer as poor communication adversely affects adjustment, treatment adherence, and potentially, survivability (Gotcher, 1993; Sherman & Simonton, 2001). While successful adjustment to cancer requires constructive discussions, often the illness brings silence to family communications. Specifically, women with cancer report being dissatisfied with the quality and quantity of communication that occurs in the family about their illness. This dissatisfaction frequently results from women having difficulty communicating about their illness and their corresponding emotional distress because they do not want to "burden" their family (Gotcher, 1993). Likewise, the family avoids initiating discussions about the illness or the woman's experience for fear of "saying the wrong thing" or upsetting her further (Gotcher, 1993; Veach et al., 2002). Ultimately, the family's difficulties communicating about the distress caused by cancer may, in part, be a function of traditional gender roles. Specifically, women traditionally serve a more communal role in families than men, and deviation from these traditional roles creates imbalance and uncertainty for both parties (Rolland, 1989).

Healthy families also use clear communication (congruence between verbal messages and metacommunication) to establish roles and boundaries between subsystems and generations (Barnhill, 1979; Nichols & Minuchin, 1999). Boundaries define and protect the integrity of these subsystems and lay the foundation for identified family roles (Vetere, 2001). Healthy families contain members who balance agency and communion, and who can demonstrate gender role flexibility in times of stress (Helgeson, 1993; 1994). Role reciprocity allows both men and women to be more central in family functioning (communion) while continuing to maintain a focus on self and personal needs (agency). In contrast, unhealthy families demonstrate rigidity in their roles characteristic of the unmitigated extremes. For example, an unmitigated agentic partner may be unable to subsume family responsibilities because of his extreme focus on himself and his personal goals. Furthermore, an unmitigated communion woman is unable to allow others to assist her with self-care, childcare, and household responsibilities because of the over-involvement with others and self-neglect characteristic of women with this trait. In contrast to those families possessing unmitigated traits, healthy families with balanced gender roles react by adjusting family roles based on appropriate shifts in responsibility, between and within generations in various life cycle stages (Carter & McGoldrick, 1989).

Family life cycle and cancer

Since women traditionally have been identified as central to the functioning of the family system and life cycle, their diagnosis with cancer places more stress on the family system and makes the family more vulnerable to disruption of normal family development (McGoldrick, 1989). Specifically, when the woman is not available to carry the burden of the family's emotional needs, due to cancer, the family may fail to accomplish the emotional processes necessary for successful transitions between life cycle or developmental stages. Successful progression through the family life cycle depends on many illness and family variables. Illness variables may include type or site of cancer, stage of cancer, course of treatment (i.e., radiation and chemotherapy), and outcome of treatment (Veach et al., 2002). The family variables of cohesion, adaptability/flexibility, communication, and family roles, discussed earlier, vary in significance depending on the life cycle stage of the family.

As the family life cycle is a model based on chronological time, it is important to note the multigenerational and parallel nature of the stages. Specifically, at a given point in time there could be three women in the multigenerational system at three different lifecycle stages coping with a woman's diagnosis of cancer. For example, the youngest woman might be in the first stage, leaving home, while her mother is in the fifth stage, launching children, and her grandmother in the final stage, families later in life. The core developmental issues at each life cycle stage will be reviewed within the context of a woman with cancer at that stage, followed by a discussion of the effect of cancer on the family at that stage. Also, the role of agency and communion will be described and implications for treatment provided at each stage.

Stage one: Leaving home. In the first stage the emphasis is on the identity processes of separation and individuation (Haley, 1997). Essentially, the young woman is working to successfully establish a balance between continuity and innovation, develop intimate peer relationships, and establish her emotional and financial independence (Carter & McGoldrick, 1999).

Women at this stage strive to develop a balance between agency or focus-on-self and communion or a sense of connectedness. Ultimately, these processes are centrifugal, such that they propel the young woman away from her family of origin while encouraging her to remain involved in social networks.

The diagnosis of cancer for a young, single woman affects her accomplishment of these life cycle tasks in three key ways. First, the diagnosis disrupts the process of establishing herself in work and intimate relationships. The centripetal force of the diagnosis often pulls the woman back into her family of origin, which is counter to the normative developmental process of separation and individuation. The more debilitating her treatment and course of illness, the more likely she will experience difficulty mastering the tasks of innovation and continuity. Second, this pull back into the family of origin may impede her successful formation of intimate peer relationships, particularly partner relationships. Finally, the young woman with cancer may be particularly vulnerable to the issues of body image and sexuality that can accompany cancer, as identity consolidation is a normative developmental task (Veach et al., 2002).

In addition, the young woman's return to her family of origin can cause disruption in other members' movement through the life cycle stages. For example, her parents' focus on her illness and recovery may interfere with their preparing her younger siblings to leave home. Her stage five parents may also invest more energy in caring for their daughter with cancer than their normative developmental task of rekindling their intimate partner bond. Finally, her return to her family of origin and reliance on them for illness care may delay her stage five mother's individuation from the family and subsequent pursuit of nonfamily interest areas.

In working with the young woman with cancer and her family, it is important to clarify the course of treatment and prognosis. Early identification of possible outcomes can help the young woman realistically appraise her expected level of independence. In cases where long-term survivability is limited, the young woman can work to establish independence within the parameters of the course of the illness. However, in cases where the prognosis is good, she can conceptualize the illness as a temporary setback in her progression through this stage.

Regardless, she should be encouraged to seek out and maintain peer relationships in order to foster developmentally appropriate emotional independence from her family of origin. These young women may grapple with accepting their post cancer appearance and sexuality, particularly with reproductive and breast cancers, as a result of feeling at odds with culturally accepted ideals. Given that identity development is part of the normative process for these young women, it is important to help them establish a healthy sense of self and an acceptance of their bodies (Veach et al., 2002).

Stage two: Joining of families through marriage. The second stage, joining of families, begins with the courtship of a new couple (Carter & McGoldrick, 1989). At this time, the couple has an idealized image of one another and they often overlook the difficulties of merging their two family systems. The new family system requires realignment of extended families and merging of finances, emotions, power, and activities (Carter & McGoldrick, 1989). Both partners in the couple negotiate a healthy balance of maintaining independence (agency) achieved at stage one with continued involvement in original and newly established social networks (communion).

When a woman is diagnosed with cancer at this stage, however, there is often an imbalance of agency and communion. For example, she may, at least temporarily, become more physically and emotionally dependent on her partner. Lewis and Hammond (1992) note that the healthy partner often reports feeling inadequate and unprepared to help the woman with cancer cope with the emotional and physical demands accompanying her cancer and its treatment. The partner often feels insecure assuming these roles in the newly emerging family system. The authors also identify that when the woman's partner had difficulty managing their own emotional reactions, making decisions, adjusting to new life responsibilities, or providing emotional support, depression increases for both the woman and partner. This depression creates greater dissatisfaction with the relationship for both. In turn, the dissatisfaction causes the woman to pull away from the newly forming relationship and move toward her family of origin, essentially resulting in a breached generational boundary. When this process occurs, the cancer serves to delay the merging of the new couple (Veach et al., 2002). When women experience greater mutuality and communion in the couple relationship, with regard to emotional experience and role adjustment, they report decreased depression and increased quality of life, self-care, and illness adjustment (Lewis & Hammond, 1992). Therefore, treatment should involve fostering mutuality and clear communication as key elements for healthy adjustment at this stage. Successful couples will maintain their connection and commitment to their relationship while also accessing extended family members for emotional and instrumental aid. Finally, mutual decisions about how to involve their families of origin in care and support of the female cancer patient will maintain the newly forming couple dyad while providing the additional resources the couple may need to cope with the illness (Patterson, 1988).

Stage three: Families with young children. In the third stage, families with young children, the focus is on acceptance of new members into the system (Carter & McGoldrick, 1989). New parents must adjust the couple dyad to accommodate their role as parents as well as partners (Aponte & VanDeusen, 1981). The new parents must make space for the child in the system and renegotiate their own roles with regard to childrearing, financial, and household tasks (Carter & McGoldrick, 1999). Typically, the changes required at this stage "combine to produce a strong shift of power . . . back toward the traditional arrangement of breadwinner dad and domestic mom" (Carter & McGoldrick, 1999, p. 254). The woman finds herself pushed to more of a communal focus than earlier stages. In contrast, the couple relationship may become more imbalanced with the partner maintaining or moving towards a more agentic focus. Successful negotiation of the increased tasks at this stage requires that new parents integrate an awareness of traditional gender roles and power imbalances often inherent in parenting young children, with the continued need for a healthy balance of agency and communion for both parents.

Little is known about the effect of cancer on the family at this time. However, the available research suggests cancer has a significant influence on the family system when the patient is a woman with young children (Lewis & Hammond, 1992). Women often are already experiencing considerable role strain within the family system at this stage. When they are diagnosed with cancer, these women experience substantial conflict between managing their family responsibilities and self-care needs, especially when other members in the system are unable or unwilling to assume increased responsibility (Kayser et al., 1999). When investigating the effect of cancer on families at this stage, Lewis and Hammond (1992) found that these mothers often report lower marital adjustment that adversely affects the overall functioning of the entire household.

Furthermore, children (ages 6-10) in the family struggle with their mother's diagnosis as evidenced by their reported fear about the integrity of the family and what might happen to them, especially if the cancer were to recur. These younger children and their older counterparts (ages 10-13) experienced sadness, fear, loneliness, worry, and occasional anger that interfered with their overall individual, social, and family functioning. Additionally, the older children's negative emotional experience appeared to adversely affect their self-esteem. Finally, the older children's social functioning was affected because they were often expected to assume new roles with increased responsibilities in order to offset disruptions to household functioning. Successful adjustment to a diagnosis of cancer at this stage involves addressing the role strain created when the woman is unable to meet both her family responsibilities and self-care needs.

Given the significant demands of parenting at this stage, it is particularly important in treatment to address the parent's role expectations within the context of gender-role socialization. Specifically, couples who demonstrate gender role flexibility will more successfully cope with the role strain created by the woman's cancer. In addition to role shifts within the couple dyad, the children can be involved in accepting developmentally appropriate increased responsibilities within the family. In order to maintain healthy development of the children, it is imperative they are not overburdened and they are encouraged to maintain normative social interaction.

Treatment with children whose mothers have cancer may need to emphasize cognitive understanding of the illness and coping with the negative emotional experiences that accompany their mother's illness. Mastery of their negative emotions can help foster healthy esteem. These children's adjustment can be further enhanced by clear communication between the couple dyad focusing on maintenance of clear generational boundaries with the children and extended family. When illness characteristics suggest the likelihood of untimely death, it is important for parents to prepare the children for impending changes in the family and to identify ways for the woman's extended family to remain involved in the children's life so they do not experience multiple losses as a result of their mother's death. Also, when the woman's death is imminent, it is important for the partners to discuss her wishes in regard to advanced directives.

Stage four: Families with adolescents. During stage four, families with adolescents, the system is working toward increasing the flexibility of family boundaries to encourage the teenager's increased agency and independence (Carter & McGoldrick, 1989). Parent-child relationships must shift to allow the teenager to "move in and out of the system." In addition, the parents begin to shift their communal focus from the children back to the couple (Carter & McGoldrick, 1989). Establishing a balance of agency and communion among all family members is an essential developmental task at this stage. In particular, the mother and adolescent children shift to identify and incorporate more agentic foci within the context of family functioning.

The woman with cancer at this stage may struggle with balancing the normative shifts in agency and communion while managing the increased demands of her medical care. For women working outside the home, cancer can affect their long-term career goals. Promoting agency around career issues will facilitate long-term adjustment for these women and maintain the sense of increased agency that is normative at this stage. For homemakers, cancer can interfere with the normative process of increasing non-childrearing interests and pursuits. While the woman with cancer at this stage will likely struggle with balancing agency and communion, the greater risk to the family system as a whole is breached generational boundaries within the family of procreation (Veach et al., 2002).

The centripetal pull of the cancer diagnosis and treatment not only influences the mother's focus away from her own increased agency, but may also pull her adolescent daughter(s) back into the system to fill both the instrumental and emotional void that can be created by their mother's illness. This process is contrary to the teen's normative centrifugal shift away from the family and toward increased agency. Older adolescent daughters may be especially vulnerable to this role strain when there are younger children in the family. Parents in these families may feel pressured to increase the daughter's responsibilities and restrict their boundaries, thereby limiting her capacity to move out of the system (Veach et al., 2002). This tendency will be especially strong in families holding traditional gender-role expectations, when these young women will be perceived as an additional resource to fill the void left by their mother. Likewise, the female daughters of women with cancer are at increased risk for incorporating unrealistic ideals for caregiving (unmitigated communion) as part of their identity as a result of the extreme influence on caring for others in their formative years. Male and female adolescents whose mother has cancer often experience esteem difficulties, specifically poor self-worth, which ultimately places an additional stress on the family system (Lewis & Hammond, 1992).

In counseling, healthy adjustment can be fostered by clarifying generational boundaries and appropriate roles, particularly with regard to adolescent daughters meeting the emotional and instrumental needs previously met by their now ill mother. Although adolescents are developmentally equipped to carry more responsibility with regard to household tasks, they should be encouraged to maintain peer and leisure involvement as much as possible regardless of gender. In order to reduce the adolescent's burden, the couple dyad can identify ways to garner support from extended family members without breaching generational boundaries. Again, communication and role flexibility between partners can serve to strengthen their relationship and enhance family system functioning.

Stage five: Launching children. The fifth stage, launching children, is the longest phase in the lifecycle and can last 20 years or more. This stage requires that families accept many entries into and exits from the family system (Carter & McGoldrick, 1989). At this stage, there is much realignment in the system as children begin to leave home and introduce new, extended family members via their union with another system. The process of realignment often requires new roles, rules, and subsystem boundaries as parents adopt adult-adult relationships with their children (Carter & McGoldrick, 1989; Veach et al., 2002). Due to the many exits at this stage, many mothers experience "the empty nest" syndrome and as a result often venture outside the family system to incorporate new, non-childcare interests and activities into their identity (Lerner, 1998). The continued shift from a family focus to a self-focus contributes to a change in the balance of agency and communion for the woman individually and within the couple dyad. This shift in focus and change in interests often creates tension in the partner relationship and subsequent couple dyad problems (Carter & McGoldrick, 1999). Healthy families use their communication skills to negotiate these role shifts and balance individual and family needs.

A diagnosis with cancer can be especially difficult in the early years of this stage for women whose primary focus has been homemaking. Her diagnosis and treatment with cancer can interfere with her continued shift away from communal family roles, toward her own personal agentic goals. For women with limited non-childcare interests and activities, the cancer may become the focus of her identity and involvement. While all women treated for cancer at this stage can experience difficulty balancing their own needs for self-care and the needs of their elder relatives, women whose primary focus has been the family may have greater difficulty striking this balance.

The diagnosis and treatment of cancer at this stage also interferes with the normative realignment of relationships between the parents and their adult children. As the woman becomes more debilitated, either because of adjuvant therapies or advanced stages of cancer, her grown children are often drawn back into the family of origin. Again daughters of mothers with cancer are more vulnerable to this pull and may experience conflict between the developmental push to exit the system and start their own family and the pull to remain a part of their family of origin (Veach et al., 2002). This pull is particularly strong for the daughters of women with cancer who exhibit unmitigated communion traits because of their tendency to return to the family of origin to assume the caregiver role for their ill mothers. When this process occurs, it exacerbates the role strain already experienced by this "sandwich generation" of women, who are working to meet the needs of their family of choice as well as the needs of their family of origin.

At this stage, encouraging the woman with cancer and her partner to utilize the resources within their couple dyad to meet her instrumental and emotional needs during her treatment and recovery will enhance healthy adjustment. She and her partner may have to creatively work together to find ways to provide care for their elder relatives without adding to the female cancer patient's role strain. Women with cancer at this stage who have not yet had significant non-childcare interests and activities should be encouraged to explore aspects of their identity beyond the family and their cancer. Further, when the women at this stage are able to promote their adult-to-adult relationships with their adult children, the two generations develop skills necessary to communicate their personal needs and subsequently devise ways to provide for the needs of all generations. For example, when the cancer patient and her adult children experience role strain, they may need to access resources within other parts of their social networks rather than predominantly relying on family members.

Stage six: Families in later life. The primary developmental task in the final stage, families in later life, involves acceptance of shifting generational roles (Carter & McGoldrick, 1989). This stage is characterized by status changes, such as retirement, and the accompanying lifestyle adjustments. One lifestyle adjustment includes financial strain, especially when there is a serious illness such as cancer. Another adjustment includes the increased amount of time partners spend with each other. Couples that have maintained a strong couple dyad throughout the parenting and launching years are able to retain a sense of agency by maintaining their own functioning in the face of physical decline while allowing and even encouraging their adult children to communally explore new family roles in separate subsystems. In addition, successful adaptation to the shrinking community of friends and relatives is facilitated when the couple dyad is strong. Overall, the focus in the aging couple system returns primarily to a communal or systems focus.

As with many life-threatening illnesses, the risk for cancer increases with age. In particular, one in three women copes with a diagnosis of cancer in later life (American Cancer Society, 2003). Schnoll and Harlow (2001) note that older cancer patients often experience less distress associated with their diagnosis because they have previously achieved many of the common developmental tasks of our society. While illness and death are normative at this stage, the woman with cancer may struggle with limited financial and personal resources to cope with the illness. Most often it is the woman's adult children who care for her during her cancer treatment and recovery. This role reversal can be difficult for both child and parent. In healthy families, the parent and adult child negotiate new boundaries such that the adult child provides support, but does not take over functioning for their ill parent (Veach et al., 2002). This role reversal is particularly difficult in traditional, communal families where the mother is perceived as the primary caregiver and emotional stronghold. In treatment, assisting these families with the typical life tasks of this stage may include having the family engage in a life review, identifying resources outside the family system, and realigning the generational roles to accommodate loss of elders.

Conclusion

Cancer affects the family system in a multitude of ways. The woman's diagnosis affects the family by forcing adjustment to new and varied roles, rules, and responsibilities. In order to cope with cancer at any given life stage, the family must fill lost roles, cope with demands of the illness, meet family members' emotional needs, and continue progression through the family life cycle. The preceding discussion highlights ways in which gender-role socialization greatly affects the adjustment of the patient and the response of her family to the changes prompted by the clinical course of cancer. Therefore, clinicians working with families affected by cancer should incorporate knowledge of gender-role socialization within the context of general systems principles and the family life cycle. These constructs have been integrated in this paper in order to provide a framework for working with female cancer patients and their families. However, it remains important to note that only a few of the many possible cancer and family scenarios are presented in the context of this paper. Ultimately, this paper strives to provide a nomothetic perspective to coping with cancer in a family consisting of a couple with children. Since variations likely exist for many patients, clinicians are encouraged to utilize the information presented in an ideographic manner to best meet any individual woman's needs.

References

Allen, S. M., & Hawkins, A. J. (1999). Maternal gatekeeping: Mothers' beliefs and behaviors that inhibit greater father involvement in family work. *Journal of Marriage and the Family, 61*, 199-212.

American Cancer Society (2003). Cancer facts and figures. Retrieved on May 22, 2003, from http://www.cancer.org/downloads/STT/CAFF2003PWSecured.pdf.

Aponte, H. J., & VanDeusen, J. M. (1981). Structural family therapy. In A. Gurman and D. P. Kniskern (Eds.), *Handbook of family therapy* (pp. 310-360). New York: Brunner/Mazel.

Bakan (1966). *The duality of human existence*. Chicago: Rand McNally.

Barnhill, L. R. (1979). Healthy family systems. *The Family Coordinator, January*, 94-100.

Bolger, N., Foster, M., Vinokur, A.D., & Ng, R. (1996). Close relationships and adjustment to a life crisis: The case of breast cancer. *Journal of Personality and Social Psychology, 70*, 283-294.

Buss, D. M. (1990). Unmitigated agency and unmitigated communion: An analysis of the negative components of masculinity and femininity. *Sex Roles, 22*, 555-568.

Carter, B., & McGoldrick, M. (1989). *The changing family lifecycle: A framework for family therapy (2nd ed.)*. Needham Heights, MA: Allyn & Bacon.

Carter, B., & McGoldrick, M. (1999). *The extended family lifecycle: Individual, family, and social perspectives (3rd ed.)*. Needham Heights, MA: Allyn & Bacon.

Freidan, B. (1997). *Beyond gender: The new politics of work and family*. Washington, D.C.: The Woodrow Wilson Center.

Fritz, H. L., & Helgeson, V. S. (1998). Distinctions of unmitigated communion from communion: Self-neglect and over-involvement with others. *Journal of Personality and Social Psychology, 75*, 121-140.

Goldenberg, I., & Goldenberg, H. (1996). *Family therapy: An overview*. Pacific Grove, CA: Brooks/Cole.

Gotcher, J. M. (1993). The effects of family communication on psychosocial adjustment of cancer patients. *Journal of Applied Communication Research, 17*, 176-188.

Haley, J. (1987). *Problem-solving therapy (2nd ed.)*. San Francisco, CA: Jossey-Bass/Pfeiffer.

Haley, J. (1997). *Leaving home: The therapy of disturbed young people (2nd ed.)*. Philadelphia: Brunner/Mazel.

Helgeson, V. S. (1993). Implications of agency and communion for patient and partner adjustment to a first coronary event. *Journal of Personality and Social Psychology, 64*, 807-816.

Helgeson, V. S. (1994). Relation of agency and communion to psychological well-being: Evidence and potential explanations. *Psychological Bulletin, 116*, 412-428.

Helgeson, V. S., & Fritz, H. L. (2000). The implications of unmitigated agency and unmitigated communion for domains of problem behavior. *Journal of Personality, 68*, 1031-1056.

Helgeson, V. S., & Lepore, S. J. (1997). Men's adjustment to prostate cancer: The role of agency and unmitigated agency. *Sex Roles, 37*, 251-267.

Jacklin, C. N. (1989). Female and male: Issues of gender. *American Psychologist, 44*, 127-133.

Jacobs, J., Ostroff, J., & Steinglass, P. (1998). Family therapy: A systems approach to cancer care. In J. Holland (Ed.), *Psycho-oncology* (pp. 994-1003). New York: Oxford University.

Kayser, K., Sormanti, M., & Strainchamps, E. (1999). Women coping with cancer: The influence of relationship factors on psychosocial adjustment. *Psychology of Women Quarterly, 23*, 725-739.

Lederberg, M. S. (1998). The family of the cancer patient. In J. Holland (Ed.), *Psycho-oncology* (pp. 981-993). New York: Oxford University.

Lerner (1998). *The mother dance*. New York, NY: Harper Collins.

Lewis, F. M., & Hammond, M. A. (1992). Psychosocial adjustment of the family to breast cancer: A longitudinal analysis. *Journal of the American Medical Women's Association, 47*, 104-200.

McCreary, D. R., & Korabik, K. (1994). Examining the relationships between the socially desirable and undesirable aspects of agency and communion. *Sex Roles, 31*, 637-651.

McGoldrick, M. (1989). Women and the family lifecycle. In B. Carter & M. McGoldrick (Eds.), *The changing family lifecycle: A framework for family therapy (2nd ed.)* (pp. 31-68). Needham Heights, MA: Allyn & Bacon.

Nicholas, D. R., & Veach, T. A. (2000). The psychosocial assessment of the adult cancer patient. *Professional Psychology: Research and Practice, 31*(2), 206-215.

Nichols, M. P., & Minuchin, S. (1998). Structural family therapy. In J. M. Donovan (Ed.), *Short-term couple therapy* (pp. 124-143). New York: Guilford.

Nichols, M. P., & Schwartz, R. C. (1995). *Family therapy: Concepts and methods (3rd ed.)*. Boston: Allyn & Bacon.

Olson, D. H. (1993). Circumplex model of marital and family systems: Assessing family functioning. In F. Walsh (Ed.), *Normal family processes*. New York: Guilford.

Olson, D. H., & Lavee, Y. (1989). Family systems and family stress: A family lifecycle perspective. In K. Kreppner & R. M. Lerner (Eds.), *Family systems and life-span development* (pp. 165-195). Hillsdale, NJ: Lawrence Erlbaum.

Patterson, J. M. (1988). Families experiencing stress: The family adjustment and adaptation response model. *Family Systems Medicine, 5*, 202-237.

Piro, M., Zeldrow, P. B., Knight, S. J., Mytko, J. J., & Gradishar, W. J. (2001). The relationship between agentic and communal personality traits and psychosocial adjustment to breast cancer. *Journal of Clinical Psychology in Medical Settings, 8*, 263-271.

Radina, M. E., & Armer, J. M. (2001). Post-breast cancer lymphedema and the family: A qualitative investigation of families coping with chronic illness. *Journal of Family Nursing, 7,* 281-299.

Rolland, J. (1998). Chronic illness and the family lifecycle. In B. Carter & M. McGoldrick (Eds.), *The changing family lifecycle: A framework for family therapy (2nd ed.)* (pp. 433-456). Needham Heights, MA: Allyn & Bacon.

Schnoll, R. A., & Harlow, L. L. (2001). Using disease-related and demographic variables to form cancer-distress risk groups. *Journal of Behavioral Medicine, 24,* 57-73.

Sherman, A. C., & Simonton, S. (2001). Coping with cancer in the family. *Family Journal: Counseling and Therapy for Couples and Families, 9,* 193-200.

Spence, J. T., Helmrich, R. L., & Holahan, C. K. (1979). Negative and positive component of psychological masculinity and femininity and their relationship to self-reports of neurotic and acting out behaviors. *Journal of Personality and Social Psychology, 37,* 1673-1682.

Veach, T. A., Nicholas, D. R., & Barton, M. A. (2002). *Cancer and the family lifecycle: A practitioner's guide.* Lillington, NC: Edwards Brothers.

Vess, J. D., Moreland, J. R., & Schwebel, A. I. (1985). A follow-up study of role functioning and the psychological environment of families of cancer patients. *Journal of Psychosocial Oncology, 3,* 1-14.

Vetere, A. (2001). Structural family therapy. *Child Psychology and Psychiatry Review, 6,* 133-139.

Vinokur, A. D., Threatt, B. A., Caplan, R. D., & Zimmerman, B. L. (1989). Physical and psychosocial functioning and adjustment to breast cancer: Long-term follow-up of a screening population. *Cancer, 63,* 394-405.

Feminist-Informed Medical Family Therapy Principles and Techniques Across Biopsychosocial Systems Levels for Younger Women with Breast Cancer and their Partners

Stephanie R. Burwell, Bowden Templeton, Kelly S. Kennedy and Lisa Zak-Hunter

ABSTRACT
Nearly one fourth of women diagnosed with breast cancer are aged 50 and younger. Little is known about the impact of diagnosis or treatment on younger women and their relationships with their spouse or partner. The purpose of this paper is to (a) describe the issues younger women with breast cancer face, (b) identify how these issues impact the relationship between younger women with breast cancer and their spouse or partner, and (c) present an integrated feminist-informed medical family therapy model to assist younger women with breast cancer and their partners during diagnosis, treatment, and transition to survivorship.

The most common type of cancer among women in the United States is breast cancer, with 178,480 new cases of breast cancer expected in 2007 (American Cancer Society, 2007). Recent attention has focused on the needs of younger women with breast cancer, as at least one fourth of newly diagnosed women are aged 50 or younger (American Cancer Society, 2001). Compared to women over 50, younger women with breast cancer generally have more problems adjusting to and coping with cancer, have higher risk of disease, undergo more aggressive treatments for breast cancer, have poorer quality of life and survival rates, and have psychosocial problems encountered less often by older women (Avis, Crawford, & Manuel, 2004; Baider et al., 2002; Cordova et al., 1995; Ganz, Rowland, Desmond, Meyerowitz, & Wyatt, 1998; Ganz, Rowland, Meyerowitz, & Desmond, 1998; King, Kenny, Shiell, Hall, & Boyages, 2000; Manuel et al., 2007; Mor, Malin, & Alien, 1994; Nixon et al., 1994; Swanson & Lin, 1994). Other problems of particular concern among younger women include family planning and infertility, as aggressive breast cancer treatments can bring about premature menopause and ovarian failure (Dow & Kuhn, 2004; Mor et al., 1994; Schover, 1999).

The psychosocial impact of a breast cancer diagnosis extends beyond the patient and can be felt throughout the family system, especially among spouses or partners (Baider et al., 2004; Ben-Zur, 2001; Compas et al., 1994; Manne, 1998; Northouse & Swain, 1987; Peteet & Greenberg, 1995; Shands, Lewis, Sinsheimer, & Cochrane, 2006), who commonly adopt caregiving roles during treatment (Northouse, 1989; Pistrang & Barker, 1995). The purpose of this paper is to (a) describe specific issues younger women with breast cancer face during diagnosis, treatment, and survivorship, as reported in the existing literature; (b) identify how these issues impact the relationship between younger women with breast cancer and their spouse or partner; and (c) present a feminist-informed medical family therapy approach to working with younger women with breast cancer and their partners during diagnosis, treatment, and survivorship using a case example.

Diagnostic phase

A woman's diagnosis of breast cancer often evokes a range of psychological reactions including fear, distress, shock, and sadness (Broom, 2001). Younger women may be especially vulnerable to disruption in quality of life compared to older women as a result of their stage in the life cycle. Younger women may be balancing multiple life demands and their corresponding roles, such as raising young children and participating in the paid workforce, while trying to adapt to and manage breast cancer diagnosis and treatment (Petersen, Kruczek, & Shaffner, 2003).

Relationship Stressors and Partner Communication

Numerous studies show that during the diagnostic phase of breast cancer, women experience high levels of psychological distress (ThomasMacLean, 2004; Northouse 1989; Wilkinson, 2001). Prior to breast biopsy, women show increased problems in daily living and levels of anxiety higher than those of acutely ill psychiatric patients (Northouse, Tocco, & West, 1997; Scott, 1983). In a cross-sectional study of 300 women and 265 of their husbands, Northouse et al. (1997) found that one week prior to biopsy, women worry about pain, disfigurement, and surgery outcome. Of these women, 38% reported the highest level of concern regardless of what their physicians told them about breast cancer diagnosis prior to biopsy. In a study of 50 couples one month post mastectomy, 83% of patients and 50% of husbands reported that, compared to breast cancer treatment and adaptation, the diagnostic phase is the most stressful (Northouse, 1989).

Fewer studies have focused on spouse and partner reactions to breast cancer. We were unable to locate any studies specifically targeting spouses or partners of younger women with breast cancer. The existing literature on partner reactions to breast cancer regardless of age suggests that husbands report levels of psychological distress similar to that of their wives (Northouse et al., 1997; Northouse, Jeffs, Cracchiolo-Caraway, Lampman, & Dorris, 1995; Peteet & Greenberg, 1995; Sabo, 1990), and feel inadequate in their ability to help their wives cope with their diagnosis (Sabo, 1990). In a qualitative study of 67 partners of women diagnosed with breast cancer within the past two and a half years, men reported feeling inadequate and unprepared for the emotional upheaval following breast cancer diagnosis. The men in this study also described wanting to protect their wives from the emotional sequelae of breast cancer (Zahlis & Shands, 1991). However, Northouse et al. (1995) found that the level of partner distress during the diagnostic phase, as measured by the Brief Symptom Inventory (Derogatis & Melisaratos, 1983), is only slightly more than that found in the normal population and less than their wives' distress level.

Sexual Relationship

Most of the research on sexual function among younger women with breast cancer has been conducted during the treatment and survivorship phases (e.g., Ganz, Rowland, Desmond, et al., 1998; Ganz, Rowland, Meyerowitz, et al., 1998; Holmberg, Scott, Alexy, & Fife, 2001; Rowland et al., 2000; Yurek, Farrar, & Anderson, 2000; Burwell, Case, Kaelin, & Avis, 2006). Few studies have focused on sexual function or the sexual relationship of younger women with breast cancer during the diagnostic phase. In a cross-sectional study of younger women with breast cancer, Bloom, Stewart, Chang, and Banks (2004) compared 167 women 1–2 months post diagnosis to 169 women 6–7 months post diagnosis and found that women in the treatment phase closer to diagnosis (1–2 months versus 6–7 months) reported a better body image. They speculated that in the early stages of disease, young women focus more on immediate survival and are less concerned about issues related to sexuality (Bloom et al., 2004).

Interactions with Physicians

For patients and their families, understanding breast cancer, its course, and its treatment can be overwhelming and complex, making physician–patient communication imperative. To date, little research has been conducted in the area of physician–patient communication among breast cancer patients, and we were unable to locate any research on the communication or specific interaction between couples and physicians. Physician–patient communication behaviors that have been studied among breast cancer patients regardless of age include interactive and tangible information giving, emotional support, and a participatory decision-making style (Maly, Leake, & Silliman, 2004; Takayama & Yamazaki, 2004). In general, women report greater satisfaction with their physician when they are able to be interactive in the discussion of diagnosis and treatment options. In a cross-sectional study of 222 older women with breast cancer, women who had more interaction with their physician showed greater knowledge about breast cancer and had shorter delay in treatment selection (Maly et al., 2004). In another cross-sectional study of 86 women with breast cancer, the patient's anxiety level predicted the perceived success associated with the interaction with their physician, suggesting that physicians who are attentive to their patient's emotional state may be more likely to have a successful interaction with their patient (Takayama & Yamazaki, 2004).

Treatment phase

Relationship Stressors and Partner Communication

Stressors placed on women and their partners during the treatment phase are significant. During chemotherapy and radiation, women commonly report fatigue, nausea, and cancer-related pain (Baron, Fey, Borgen, & Van Zee, 2004; Harmer, 2006; Hordern, 2000; Wilmoth, Coleman, Smith, & Davis, 2004). As a result, partners of women with breast cancer find themselves taking on greater household, parenting, and caregiving responsibilities (Vess, Moreland, Schwebel, & Kraut, 1988). These role shifts can place great strain on the couple as they adjust to breast cancer (Northouse, Templin, Mood, & Oberst, 1998). In a study examining psychosocial adjustment to a recent breast cancer diagnosis among 111 mothers, depression was linked to the mother's amount of increased role responsibilities following diagnosis (Lewis & Hammond, 1992). In a landmark longitudinal study, Vess, Moreland, and Schwebel (1985a,1985b) found that spousal communication patterns and cohesion or conflict in the family strongly predicted the extent to which certain roles were retained among 54 couples.

Following breast cancer diagnosis, communication between women and their partners may become strengthened or more problematic. Maintaining or increasing communication between couples adjusting to cancer has many positive effects including increased intimacy and connection (Burwell, Brucker, & Shields, 2006; Manne, Ostroff, Rini, et al., 2004). However, communication problems may become exacerbated in relationships where problems existed prior to breast cancer diagnosis. In some cases, a diagnosis of breast cancer serves as an impetus for a patient or partner to leave a troubled or unhappy relationship (Holmberg et al., 2001; Walsh, Manuel, & Avis, 2005). In other cases couples are able to communicate well for the most part but experience difficulty discussing specific issues, particularly death and dying, and fears related to having cancer (Petersen et al., 2003; Shands et al., 2006; Walsh et al., 2005).

Younger women have reported that communication avoidance and other communication problems place strain on their relationship with their partner (Walsh et al., 2005) and negatively affect their adjustment to illness (Manne, Taylor, Dougherty, & Kemeny, 1997). In a study of 148 breast cancer patient couples, Manne et al. (2004) had couples watch a video of a dyad communicating about breast cancer and measured their reactions using the Rapid Marital Interaction Coding System (Heyman & Vivian, 1997). They found that patients reported significantly less distress when partners self-disclosed and were less likely to offer solutions. Manne et al. (2006) also examined cancer-related communication in 147 patients and 127 partners, and found that demand-withdraw and mutualwithdraw behaviors in couples were significantly associated with worse relationship satisfaction, whereas couples' mutually constructive communication was associated with better relationship satisfaction.

Spouses and partners of women with breast cancer must also cope with the impact the illness will have on the lives of their family (Manne, 1998; Manne et al., 2006; Manne, Sherman, et al., 2004; Northouse, Templin, & Mood, 2001; Shands et al., 2006; Wagner, Bigatti, & Storniolo, 2006). Often the spouse or partner is forgotten during breast cancer treatment and may find it difficult to communicate about the illness. Friends, family, and other members of the patient's support network may realize the impact of the illness on the patient but overlook the partner's concerns and fears. Partners may believe that communicating about breast cancer is detrimental or burdensome to the patient and internalize their concerns and feelings to protect their partner (Petersen et al., 2003). However, in a study of 98 women with breast cancer and their partners, patient disclosure and partner disclosure and responsiveness were found to lead to higher levels of intimacy when compared to couples who did not disclose feelings (Manne, Ostroff, Rini, et al., 2004).

Sexual Relationship

The couple's sexual relationship appears to suffer the most during the treatment phase. Breast cancer treatments such as chemotherapy, radiation, and endocrine therapy have been shown to be associated with fatigue, decrease in sexual interest and desire, menopausal symptoms, vaginal dryness, and diminished sexual response in younger women (Burwell et al., 2006; Ganz, Desmond, Belin, Meyerowitz, & Rowland, 1999; Ganz, Greendale, Petersen, Kahn, & Bower, 2003; Ganz, Rowland, Desmond, et al., 1998; Ganz, Rowland, Meyerowitz, et al., 1998; Greendale, Petersen, Zibecchi, & Ganz, 2001; Harmer, 2006; Holmberg et al., 2001). Younger women are particularly worried about being rejected by their partner as a result of disfigurement due to mastectomy (Henson, 2002), and it is not surprising that greater sexual dysfunction occurs following mastectomy than breast conservation surgery (Harmer, 2006; Henson, 2002). In a cross-sectional study of 1,957 breast cancer survivors, approximately 40% of women who underwent mastectomy (with or without reconstruction) experienced negative sexual effects (Rowland et al., 2000). The decrease in sexual activity among mastectomy patients may be explained not only by the physical weakness and fatigue women experience following surgery but also by what the surgery symbolizes. In Western cultures, femininity is often associated with a woman's breasts. Some women have difficulty with their sexuality and perceived femininity following surgical alteration. For example, women who place more importance on the appearance and sensation of their breasts are more likely to have postoperative sexual problems (Northouse, 1994; Schain, d'Angelo, Dunn, Lichter, & Pierce, 1994; Vess et al., 1988a, 1988b).

Compared to older women, younger women in committed relationships are more likely to choose reconstructive surgery following mastectomy (Rowland et al., 2000). Compared to women who undergo lumpectomy and mastectomy without reconstruction, women who have breast reconstruction surgery tend to exhibit more postoperative sexual avoidance and situational distress, diminished sexual responsiveness and arousal, and sexual embarrassment 1 to 3 months after surgery (Yurek et al., 2000). Over time, reconstructive surgery may protect a women's body image but not her positive sexual adjustment (Henson, 2002; Yurek et al., 2000). Some women report that the reconstructed breast or breasts does or do not look like the existing (or previous) breast or breasts (Henson, 2002). A woman may mourn the loss of her breast(s), and husbands may not be able to accept the new breast(s) or surgical scarring (Nissen, Swensen, & Kina, 2002). Women whose husbands are more willing to look at and discuss the new breast(s) soon after surgery tend to adjust better than those whose husbands are avoidant (Wilmoth et al., 2004). Furthermore, when the sexual partner is emotionally involved, greater sexual, martial, and emotional adjustments occur (Wimberly, Carver, Laurenceau, Harris, & Antoni, 2005).

In a recent review of the literature, Bakewell and Volker (2005) found that a woman's perceived degree of social support and the nature of her relationships with others prior to diagnosis were the strongest predictors of long-term sexual adjustment to breast cancer. Women who were in supportive, intimate relationships had better long-term adjustment. As husbands initially fear the potential loss and death of their partner, emphasis on the sexual relationship immediately diminishes following diagnosis (Holmberg et al., 2001). Husbands have reported that the health of their spouse is more important than sex (Holmberg et al., 2001), and sexual interest also decreases among husbands who fear they may hurt their wives during sex (Northouse, 1994). Further, Northouse (1994) found that 25%–33% of married couples experience sexual difficulties related to breast cancer diagnosis, and the risk of sexual difficulties increases if these difficulties precede diagnosis.

Interactions with Physicians

While there are few studies addressing the relationship between breast cancer patients, partners, and their physicians, women undergoing treatment have described these interactions informally on breast cancer Web sites and blogs. Notable exceptions are Pitts's (2004) content analysis of 50 Web pages of women with breast cancer and Orgad's (2005) qualitative study of 41 women who used cancer-related Web sites. A predominant theme throughout both studies was that women and their partners had difficulty understanding the diagnosis and treatment options and felt intimidated, ignorant, or both at times when talking to health care providers about breast cancer (Orgad, 2005; Pitts, 2004).

In another qualitative study, 12 women were interviewed about their memories of breast cancer treatment and described feeling detached from the physician who provided their treatment (Thomas-MacLean, 2004). Some of these women felt that their physicians did not care about them and avoided becoming emotionally involved in their treatment. Some theorized that their physicians were emotionally distant as a way to deal with the pain and suffering generally related to treating patients with life-threatening disease. Women often felt unheard, unsupported, and even powerless when their physician did not attend to their concerns. They may also feel scared or helpless when their physician, who is in a position of power, views them as another case instead of engaging in a more personal interaction (ThomasMacLean, 2004). At the same time, it is also important to be mindful of the challenges health care providers face, especially given the time constraints imposed by managed care. Physicians are not afforded much time to spend with patients or their families. This tension clearly plays a role in the treatment of disease and impacts the patient and her spouse or partner.

It is not uncommon for women and their partners to feel overwhelmed by breast cancer treatments (Orgad, 2005; Pitts, 2004; Shands et al., 2006) and at times wonder if the physician's treatment recommendation is the best option for them. In Pitts's (2004) study analyzing 50 breast cancer patients' personal Web pages, one theme implied that even when physicians attempt to explain treatment options and possible side effects, many patients do not feel that they have received enough information or are empowered to choose their course of treatment (Meyer, Russo, & Talbot, 1995; Pitts, 2004). Meyer et al. examined 94 women with breast cancer and their decision-making process and found that younger women sought more information regarding treatment and took longer to decide what treatment option would be right for them. This "wait time" often raises concern in physicians who need to aggressively treat the cancer and do not want their patients to get lost in an overburdened treatment system. In addition, women may have trouble asking another physician for a second opinion about treatment options. In a study by Shands et al. (2006), 29 couples were interviewed about their core concerns about dealing with breast cancer. A main finding was that couples wanted to understand their options from different perspectives before making a treatment decision (Shands et al., 2006).

Survivorship

According to the American Cancer Society (2001), survivorship is defined as living five years beyond cancer diagnosis. Other cancer organizations have adopted this time frame as a reference for defining survivorship. However, several studies use treatment completion as a marker of survivorship and are described below (Damush, Perkins, & Miller, 2006; Rabin & Pinto, 2006; Rabin, Pinto, Trunzo, Frierson, & Bucknam, 2006).

Relationship Stressors and Partner Communication

Social context and social support are considered two of the most important factors that determine how well women with breast cancer adjust to their role as survivors (Weiss, 2004a, 2004b; Lewis et al., 2001). Social support can help curtail the lasting side effects of breast cancer among long-term survivors (Lewis et al., 2001). Spouses and partners often serve as the primary source of social support and greatly influence social context. Partners who are supportive are in a position to help breast cancer survivors deal with a range of emotional responses as they progress through the diagnostic, treatment, and survivorship phases. In fact, decreases in patient psychological distress are seen when spouses offer open and empathic communication (Pistrang & Barker, 1995).

Weiss (2004a, 2004b) studied posttraumatic growth (PTG) among 72 breast cancer survivors and their husbands. Posttraumatic growth refers to "positive views of self, sense of relationship with others, and philosophy of life" (Weiss, 2004b, p. 733). Weiss found that marital support and a positive, affective family climate are significant predictors of posttraumatic growth (Weiss, 2004b). These data also suggest that husbands' growth was significantly related to general social support, positive marital qualities, and their wives' PTG levels (Weiss, 2004a). It appears that the nature of the relationship is recursive, as women who have supportive husbands experience more PTG, and men whose wives experience more PTG have higher PTG levels themselves (Weiss, 2004a; Weiss, 2004b).

However, not all women receive support from their partner, and the relationship itself can be a source of stress (Manne, 1999; Manne, Alfieri, Taylor, & Dougherty, 1999; Shields & Rousseau, 2004). Communication problems among cancer survivors and their partners are not uncommon (Walsh et al., 2005; Shields & Rousseau, 2004). Survivors who are unable to communicate about their cancer experience with their significant other may struggle to process the event themselves. This can lead to increased psychological distress (Manne, 1999). Therefore, it is imperative that survivors and their partners learn to openly communicate about their breast cancer experience.

During the course of the illness, younger women may find that their communication patterns with their partner lead to feeling more connected or further distanced from them. On the one hand, they may find that the illness dominates communication in the relationship and that they are drawn closer as a result. On the other hand, the couple may feel distant because of the distress and fear the illness imposes on the relationship. Many individuals forget, however, that the patient *and* the partner must manage the impact of breast cancer, especially concerns related to family and work responsibilities, boundary setting, and roles that may have shifted as a result of breast cancer (Rolland, 1994b). Once a woman has reached survivorship status, family roles or responsibilities that initially shifted in response to breast cancer may return to the status quo (Petersen et al., 2003).

Sexual Relationship

As younger women become survivors, long-term effects from treatment can continue to impair their sexual function and relationship. Some of these effects are permanent, such as premature menopause (Ganz, Rowland, Desmond, et al., 1998; Schover, 1994). These biological processes can affect sexual desire, arousal, interest, and activity (Ganz et al., 1999; Ganz et al., 2003; Ganz, Rowland, Desmond, et al., 1998; Ganz, Rowland, Meyerowitz, et al., 1998; Greendale et al., 2001; Hartman, 2004). From a relational perspective, some women feel their emotional needs are not being met by a partner and therefore have no desire or interest to engage in sexual activity (Walsh et al., 2005). Some women report that they do not feel whole following mastectomy (Hartman, 2004), and others are not sure whether to conceal their surgical scars or show them to their partner (Wilkinson, 2001), which impacts multiple domains of sexual function and sexuality in general.

Some women have difficulty developing a sense of personal agency following the surgical removal of one or both breasts. A study examining Web pages of breast cancer patients found that women believed the Internet to be an empowering resource where they could share stories about losing one or both breasts while trying to make sense of incompatible cultural sexual norms. In this forum, women used humor, poetry, and journaling to express their concerns and describe the challenges and changes they experienced related to their sexuality (Pitts, 2004).

Interactions with Physicians

The label "survivor" does not imply that the breast cancer patient has completed all aspects of treatment. Survivors continue to interact with physicians for wellness checks and, in some cases, continued medication management, particularly women undergoing hormone therapies. Some patients and partners feel better equipped to understand continued medication use or physician visits by exploring the Internet or other resources. Exposure to and comprehension of the amount of information available may help a couple decide upon the best course of long-term management and surveillance. Often physicians hand a patient a prescription that she does not fully understand despite the increase in literature about medications and their side effects (Pitts, 2004). For example, some women undergo hormone treatments that often have side effects, and some couples feel they are not adequately informed to make choices about continued medication use (Pitts, 2004). Many women have also stated that they felt lost or abandoned after their acute or primary treatment ended. In a qualitative study (Thomas-MacLean, 2004), women said that they did not know where to go for information or help after their immediate treatment ended. Many times they had questions, but their physicians were not easily accessible and they did not visit with them as often.

Feminist-informed medical family therapy

In its broadest context, feminism is a lens through which we can contextualize the social and cultural construction and analysis of gender and power. In general, feminism attends to the oppression and subordination of marginalized

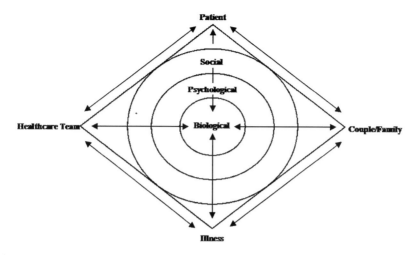

FIGURE 1 Interconnections across biopsychosocial levels and the treatment system.

populations based on gender, race, class, sexual orientation, and age (Baber & Allen, 1992). We propose that the use of a feminist framework in medical family therapy, and specifically oncology, may allow for a more inclusive explanation of the roles that gender and power play among healthcare providers, patients, and their families.

Over the past two decades, an increasing body of literature has indicated a need for collaboration between mental health and medical providers to offer comprehensive patient care (Blount & Bayona, 1994; Doherty & Baird, 1983; McDaniel & Cole-Kelly, 2003; McDaniel, Hepworth, & Doherty, 1992; Rolland, 1994a, 1994b; Seaburn, Lorenz, Gunn, Gawinski, & Mauksch, 2003; Walsh & Fortner, 2002). Medical family therapy is a global approach that refers to the "biopsychosocial treatment of individuals and families who are dealing with medical problems" (McDaniel et al., 1992, p. 2). In addition to collaboration with medical professionals, medical family therapists conceptualize symptoms and issues from a biopsychosocial perspective, acknowledging that all problems include biological, psychological, and social systems levels (see Figure 1). Because cancer diagnosis, treatment, and survivorship reaches beyond the patient and impacts the entire family, there is an increasing need for medical family therapy interventions in oncology.

We propose feminist-informed medical family therapy (FIMedFT) as a unique perspective from which to view and treat the demands of illness in families. The addition of a feminist lens to the practice of medical family therapy emphasizes the influence of gender and power on the treatment of and adjustment to illness. In many Western societies, the culture of medicine presupposes that the biomedical perspective is dominant and therefore privileges those who espouse this epistemology. We propose that while this biomedical perspective is absolutely necessary, it is not sufficient. We seek to practice from a perspective that honors multiple epistemologies.

Congruent with traditional medical family therapy, feminist-informed medical family therapists (FIMedFTs) are interested in working at all levels of the treatment system, including the patient, family, and health care team or system. FIMedFTs are trained in the basic biological processes involved in specific diseases and seek to understand how they impact psychological, relational, and social aspects of illness (KnudsonMartin, 2003). They are also trained to work with systems to facilitate collaboration and communication and to change interactional patterns across multiple systems levels. Below is a description of an integrated feminist medical family therapy model applied to a case example of a younger woman with breast cancer and her partner.

Case Study

"Nancy" is a 32-year-old married, white female diagnosed with stage II breast cancer. Following diagnosis, she underwent a bilateral mastectomy with immediate reconstruction. She later learned that the cancer had spread to a lymph node and was treated with chemotherapy, consisting of Adriamiacin, Cytoxin, and Taxol. She reported numerous side effects from the treatments, including vomiting, diarrhea, hair loss, discoloration of fingernails and toenails, hot flashes, night sweats, lethargy, memory loss, and lack of sex drive. The cancer was estrogen receptor positive, and Nancy was treated with antihormone therapy consisting of shots to "shut down" her ovaries and reduce the amount of estrogen in her body. Because of her BRCA mutations, she had a 60% risk for developing ovarian cancer. Nancy and her husband, "Billy*," had to make a difficult decision about whether or not she should remove her ovaries. Although they have a 4-year-old daughter, they had planned on having more children. After much consideration, Nancy and Billy agreed that she would undergo an oophorectomy (ovary removal) to reduce the threat of cancer recurrence. Nancy and Billy met with her oncologist, "Dr. Jones," and a medical family therapist, "Dr. Smith." The application of the feminist principals and techniques of the FIMedFT model applied by Dr. Smith and outlined in Table 1 are presented below.

Solicit the Illness Story from the Patient and Partner

One of the first tasks of the feminist-informed medical family therapist is to solicit the illness story or stories from the patient and family (McDaniel et al., 1992; Rolland, 1994a). Equally important in this model is consideration of the engendered psychological and social dimensions of how disease is *experienced* (Kleinman, 1988). Though each family member's experience with the illness may be different, all are important. Illness stories do not have a definitive way of being formed or told. According to Frank (1997), illness stories are created and shared with others and are not solely focused on recalling the facts of the illness. Illness stories are dynamic and continually shaped. For instance, when a

---

* Billy is a pseudonym.

TABLE 1 Feminist-informed medical family therapy principles and techniques across biopsychosocial systems levels for younger women with breast cancer and their partners

Levels	Domains	Feminist Principles	Feminist-Informed Medical Family Therapy Techniques
Biological	Genetics and genetic testing	Women are concerned about passing BC on to their daughters.	Attend to issues of gender and power. Recognize the biological dimension.
	Surgery type: Lumpectomy, mastectomy, reconstruction	Potential disfigurement can change the way one sees herself as a woman contradicting the dominant cultural view of beauty.	
	Biological changes due to treatment: Side effects	Women experience detrimental side effects that lead to feeling marginalized and powerless over their bodies and the disease.	Respect defenses, work through blame, and accept unacceptable feelings.
	Reproductive system	Women struggle with infertility problems that can effect role identity and challenge cultural expectations of women.	Be aware of and normalize developmental issues.
	Endocrine system	Chemotherapy can induce premature menopause resulting in hormonal shifts and fertility problems.	
Psychological	Body image	Cultural expectations and stereotypes related to body image affect women and their partners.	Attend to issues of gender and power.
	Mental health correlates	Women and their partners cope with depression, anxiety, illness adjustment, acceptance and uncertainty.	Solicit the illness story from the patient *and* partner.
	Identity	Becoming a patient or a caregiver influences identity development and role responsibilities.	Be aware of and normalize developmental issues.
Social	Relational distress	Engendered cultural expectations influence perceptions of diagnosis, treatment-related decision making, role strain, sexuality, parenting, and social support.	Attend to issues of gender and power. Solicit the illness story from the patient *and* her partner.
	Communication: Couple communication	Men stereotypically are socialized to protect women and are afraid to share feelings about breast cancer. Women and men experience communication avoidance, especially related to death, dying, and other topics.	Respect defenses, workthrough blame, and accept unacceptable feelings.
	Physician-patient Communication	The medical culture privileges physician perspectives, resulting in a rigid hierarchical treatment system that marginalizes patients and families.	Encourage couples to maintain communication with each other.
	Role shifts	Cultural and gender norms are challenged as couples respond to changing roles and responsibilities in and out of the home.	Be aware of and normalize developmental issues.
	Family life cycle	Younger age forces women and men to meet illness demands "off time" and necessitates reassessment of individual and family life cycle tasks.	Facilitate open communication between the family and healthcare systems.
	Navigation of the healthcare system	Lack of agency, empowerment, and access to resources makes navigating the healthcare system difficult for couples.	Keep an open-door policy. Increase agency in the patient and partner.

woman discontinues treatment for breast cancer, the illness story continues to evolve (Frank, 1997; Kleinman, 1988).

When soliciting an illness story, it is imperative to ask women and their partners questions about life before breast cancer. This can help the FIMedFT understand the extent to which breast cancer has infiltrated the couple's life. Once this context is established, the therapist can invite the couple to discuss their experiences with breast cancer (McDaniel et al., 1992). Frank (1997) discusses three specific types of illness narratives that include the (a) restitution narrative, (b) chaos narrative, and (c) quest narrative. The restitution narrative focuses on healing the body by seeking proper medical care and surviving the breast cancer. The chaos narrative reflects a lack of structure, order, reflection, and control, which fuels anxiety and inhibits communication about the illness. The quest narrative is characterized by advocacy, awareness, and telling of the story, and there is recognition that illness is a social problem, not a personal problem.

Many factors influence the illness narrative, including stage of cancer, family illness history, values, morals, personal experiences, gender, power, culture, characteristics of the couple's relationship prior to diagnosis, and available resources to manage disease. It is possible for the patient and partner to have separate illness narratives while sharing a mutual narrative. In this particular case, Nancy and Billy had different types of narratives (quest and restitution, respectively). It is important for the couple to hear each other's stories to foster compassion and validation of each unique experience.

Respect Defenses, Work Through Blame, and Accept Unacceptable Feelings

When soliciting the illness story, it is important to meet people where they are by respecting defenses, working through blame, and accepting unacceptable feelings. The FIMedFT approach places emphasis on respecting the feelings and various coping styles patients and partners experience in relation to breast cancer. At diagnosis, Nancy was initially overwhelmed with fear, anxiety, confusion, and anger, and at times she experienced a sense of numbness. She described feeling as though her body was being treated as an object, particularly in regard to her breasts and ovaries that awaited surgical removal. Nancy was concerned about disfigurement and fertility and felt powerless over her body. Billy had difficulty tolerating the intensity of Nancy's feelings and tried to encourage her to "forget about it and take charge." His tendency to problem solve interfered with his ability to be emotionally present. Dr. Smith normalized each of their reactions and provided examples of the range of feelings to be expected following the diagnosis of a life threatening illness such as breast cancer. Nancy's sense of numbness and Billy's problem-solving orientation were reframed as healthy and normal attributes that protected them from getting overwhelmed by the impact of a life threatening illness, especially disfigurement and temporary disability as a result of cancer treatment.

The couple's natural desire for control over the illness resulted in feelings of blame. In working with Drs. Smith and Jones, Nancy and Billy explored the biomedical etiology of breast cancer along with the personal meaning they attached to its onset and potential outcome. They began to manage the uncertainty of the illness, and it became clearer that their search for answers was a normal process that often remains unresolved but becomes more tolerable over time. At this point, Billy was able to better understand Nancy's feeling of loss of control over her body, as he felt that the illness had power over him, too. Both were encouraged to use these mutual feelings to their advantage by battling the illness together rather than independently.

Encourage Couples to Maintain Communication with Each Other

FIMedFTs are trained to facilitate communication and work with interactional patterns across systems levels. Though Nancy and Billy prided themselves on the open communication typical of their relationship before cancer, the stressors resulting from diagnosis created specific challenges for them. Both sensed fear, apprehension, and anger in the other but were too overwhelmed by their own experience and consequently withdrew. Further intensifying the conflict in their pattern of interaction, they argued over their different beliefs regarding the most appropriate course of treatment. Billy had a problem-solving orientation and was primarily focused Nancy's health. While Nancy was obviously concerned about her health, she was grieving the anticipated loss of her breasts, ovaries, and normal day-to-day function following surgery.

From the outset, Dr. Smith worked with Nancy and Billy to restore the open communication that had characterized their relationship prior to the diagnosis of breast cancer. The couple consequently strengthened their "we" approach to combating the illness. In addition to enhancing couple communication, Nancy and Billy were encouraged to discuss topics that were difficult with multiple family members, including their daughter and parents. Family therapy sessions created opportunities for discussion about cancer and its impact on their child, parents, siblings, and important friends that were major members of the couple's support network. Specific conversations were held with various groupings of family members about their fears, unacceptable feelings, overprotection of Nancy, role shifts, family responsibilities, issues of closeness and intimacy, sexuality, and future planning for finances through wills and powers of attorney.

Increase Agency in the Patient and Partner

Finding or maintaining a sense of agency in the context of healthcare can be difficult for breast cancer patients and their partners. Initially, Nancy and Billy were intimidated by the healthcare system and reluctant to ask questions and discuss breast cancer treatments. Dr. Smith recommended literature and online resources to help the couple become more familiar and comfortable with medical language and advised them to write down a list of questions to ask Dr. Jones at Nancy's next appointment. Dr. Smith encouraged Nancy to become involved with a local breast cancer support group, which can help patients develop and strengthen their sense of agency (Orgad, 2005). In addition to support groups (or if local support groups are not available), online message boards, blogs, and chat rooms can provide readily available forums for patients and partners to discuss breast cancer, ask questions, and receive support from others.

To increase Billy's agency, he was encouraged to be actively involved in meeting the familial demands of breast cancer by assuming appropriate roles. Billy's efforts to find his place in the healthcare system resulted in accompanying Nancy to appointments and finding out information. When Nancy felt fatigued from her treatments, Billy acted as her advocate during appointments by making sure her questions were asked and by taking notes. Billy also adopted the role of messenger for the family, relaying information about Nancy's condition and treatment to extended family and friends when she was unable.

Recognize the Biological Dimension

The foundation of the FIMedFT model is grounded in the biological dimension of illness. Drs. Jones and Smith met with Nancy and Billy to explain the disease process, prognosis, and course of breast cancer. During these visits, conversation was facilitated between the couple and healthcare providers to exchange information and answer questions. A significant biological concern that the couple had was that their young daughter would eventually be at risk for developing breast cancer. Although each partner worried about this possibility, it had remained a secret. Nancy was extremely guilt ridden as the genetic carrier, and Billy deliberately avoided this topic to protect Nancy's feelings. The secrecy around this fear was addressed in the couple relationship and also with the healthcare team so that open discussions about surveillance and genetic testing could take place.

Attend to Issues of Gender and Power

One of the major contributions of the FIMedFT model is increased attention to the role of gender and power in the treatment system. It is important to recognize that the patient, the family members, and the healthcare team are involved in care. Because the biomedical perspective is dominant in medicine, there is unspoken governance that privileges physicians' and other healthcare providers' perspectives, making it difficult to question or challenge unilateral decision making as a patient or family member. Yet, like many caring physicians, Dr. Jones wanted to share decision making and responsibility for Nancy's healthcare with her and other family members (Northouse & Northouse, 1987).

Nancy described feeling as though her body, especially her breasts, was being treated as a separate entity by her healthcare providers. She felt that the system of care did not understand or allow the opportunity to discuss the impact that losing a breast (and eventually ovaries) had on her personally as a young woman. Billy felt "caught in the middle" with Nancy, who was trying to work through feelings related to breast and ovary removal, and her physician, who was recommending treatments to save her life and prevent recurrence. Dr. Smith attended the oncology visit so that Nancy, Billy, and Dr. Jones could hear one another's perspectives, and eventually a shared understanding was obtained and expectations were clarified. In turn, this fostered a sense of agency and communion, the hallmarks of traditional medical family therapy models (McDaniel et al., 1992), which transcended systems levels.

Normalize Developmental Issues

Normalizing developmental issues is especially important for younger women with breast cancer and their partners. At age 32, Nancy was already having difficulty balancing her career with being a mother and wife. A diagnosis of breast cancer was not something she expected, especially at this stage in her life. Nancy was forced to concentrate on caring for herself when she would have normally focused her energy on her career and family. Billy had to assume additional household and childcare responsibilities and was concerned about being able to manage these demands while meeting their financial needs. Because of the medical bills and Nancy's need to miss work to receive treatments, their finances were strained. Even though the family had health insurance, it did not fully cover Nancy's medical expenses.

Another major developmental concern for Nancy and Billy was that the oophorectomy shattered their plan to eventually conceive more children, which became a focal point of numerous discussions. Although adoption was not something they considered prior to diagnosis, it became an option as a result of breast cancer treatment. Finally, one of the important developmental tasks normally associated with a younger couple is establishing itself as separate from families of origin (Carter & McGoldrick, 1989; Carter & McGoldrick, 1999). However, at times Nancy and Billy needed help from their parents to meet daily demands, and this came at a time when Nancy's aging parents anticipated needing assistance from *her*. Dr. Smith invited Nancy's parents to attend some sessions to address family needs, which included conversations about Nancy getting "sick" before her parents, which was not anticipated.

Facilitate Open Communication Between the Family and Healthcare System

Facilitating meetings for patients, family members, physicians, and other health care providers is needed to promote the sharing of information and development of treatment plans to cultivate a multidisciplinary team approach in the management of breast cancer. Dr. Smith met on several occasions with Nancy, Billy, Dr. Jones, and members of the nursing staff to create opportunities for communication and mutual understanding. As Nancy's treatment progressed, extended family members grew increasingly more comfortable with her medical care as they sought answers to questions and developed relationships with Dr. Jones and other medical staff.

Keep an Open-Door Policy

At the conclusion of treatment, patients, partners, family members, and the health care team have shared an intense personal experience in the care and management of breast cancer. New uncertainties arise about what the future holds without the continued support of medical professionals, as women and their spouses have anecdotally reported feelings of abandonment once the initial treatment for breast cancer is over. Nancy and Billy were encouraged to anticipate concerns they were likely to experience in the coming months. Dr. Smith reassured them that she was available as a resource and that she was in regular contact with Dr. Jones should they have concerns or want to "check in." This open-door policy also applied to members of the healthcare team to debrief about providing care to distressed oncology patients and their families.

Summary

The impact of breast cancer diagnosis and treatment is experienced throughout the family system. This paper highlighted particular problems that are often experienced by younger women with breast cancer and how these problems impact the relationships between younger women and their spouse or partner. Feminist-informed medical family therapy principals were outlined and applied to a case example to help guide healthcare professionals as they provide care for younger women with breast cancer and their partners.

References

American Cancer Society (2001). *Breast cancer facts and figures*. Atlanta.

American Cancer Society (2007). *Breast cancer facts and figures*. Atlanta.

Avis, N. E., Crawford, S., & Manuel, J. C. (2004). Psychosocial problems among younger women with breast cancer. *Psycho-Oncology, 12*, 1–14.

Baber, K., & Allen, K. (1992). *Women and families: Feminist reconstructions*. New York: Guilford Press.

Baider, L., Andritsch, E., Goldzweig, G., Uziely, B., Ever-Hadani, P., Hofman, G., et al. (2004). Changes in psychological distress of women with breast cancer in long-term remission and their husbands. *Psychosomatics, 45*, 58–68.

Bakewell R. T., & Volker, D. L. (2005). Sexual dysfunction related to the treatment of young women with breast cancer. *Clinical Journal of Oncology Nursing, 9*(6), 697–702.

Baron, R. H., Fey, J. V., Borgen, P. I., & Van Zee, K. J. (2004). Eighteen sensations after breast cancer surgery: A two-year comparison of sentinel lymph node biopsy and axillary lymph node dissection. *Oncology Nursing Forum, 31*, 691–698.

Ben-Zur, H. (2001). Your coping strategy and my distress: Inter-spouse perceptions of coping and adjustment among breast cancer patients and their spouses. *Families, Systems, & Health, 19*, 83–94.

Bloom, J. R., Stewart, S. L., Chang, S., & Banks, P. J. (2004). Then and now: Quality of life of young breast cancer survivors. *Psycho-Oncology, 13,* 147–160.

Blount, A., & Bayona, J. (1994). Toward a system of integrated primary care. *Family Systems Medicine, 12*(2), 171–182.

Broom, D. (2001). Reading breast cancer: Reflections on a dangerous intersection. *Health, 5,* 249–268.

Burwell, S. R., Brucker, P. S., & Shields, C. G. (2006). Attachment behaviors and proximity-seeking in cancer patients and their partners. *Journal of Couple and Relationship Therapy, 5*(3), 1–16.

Burwell, S. R., Case, D., Kaelin, C., & Avis, N. E. (2006). Sexual problems in younger women after breast cancer surgery. *Journal of Clinical Oncology, 24,* 2815–2821.

Carter, E. A., & McGoldrick, M. (1989). *The changing family life cycle: A framework for family therapy.* New York: Allyn and Bacon.

Carter, E. A., & McGoldrick, M. (1999). *The expanded family life cycle: Individual, family, and social perspectives.* New York: Allyn and Bacon.

Compas, B. E., Worsham, N. L., Epping-Jordan, J., Grant, K. E., Mireault, G., Howell, D. C., et al. (1994). When mom or dad has cancer: Markers of psychological distress in cancer patients, spouses and children. *Health Psychology, 13,* 507–515.

Cordova, M. J., Andrykowski, M. A., Kenady, D. E., McGrath, P. C., Sloan, D. A., & Redd, W. H. (1995). Frequency and correlates of posttraumatic-stress-disorder-like symptoms after treatment for breast cancer. *Journal of Consulting and Clinical Psychology, 63*(6), 981–986.

Damush, T. M., Perkins, A., & Miller, K. (2006). The implementation of an oncologist referred, exercise self-management program for older breast cancer survivors. *PsychoOncology, 15,* 884–890.

Derogatis, L. R., & Melisaratos, N. (1983). The Brief Symptom Inventory: An introductory report. *Psychological Medicine, 13,* 595–605.

Doherty, W. J., & Baird, M. A. (1983). *Family therapy and family medicine: Toward the primary care of families.* New York: Guilford Press.

Dow, K. H., & Kuhn, D. (2004). Fertility options in young breast cancer survivors: A review of the literature. *Oncology Nursing Forum, 31,* 46–53.

Frank, A. W. (1997). *The wounded storyteller: Body, illness, and ethics.* Chicago: University of Chicago Press.

Ganz, P. A., Desmond, K. A., Belin, T. R., Meyerowitz, B. E., & Rowland, J. H. (1999). Predictors of sexual health in women after a breast cancer diagnosis. *Journal of Clinical Oncology, 17,* 2371–2380.

Ganz, P. A., Greendale, G. A., Petersen, L., Kahn, B., & Bower, J. E. (2003). Breast cancer in younger women: Reproductive and late health effects of treatment. *Journal of Clinical Oncology, 21,* 4184–4193.

Ganz, P. A., Rowland, J. H., Desmond, K., Meyerowitz, B. E., & Wyatt, G. E. (1998). Life after breast cancer: Understanding women's health-related quality of life and sexual functioning. *Journal of Clinical Oncology, 16,* 501–514.

Ganz, P. A., Rowland, J. H., Meyerowitz, B. E., & Desmond, K. A. (1998). Impact of different adjuvant therapy strategies on quality of life in breast cancer survivors. *Recent Results Cancer Research, 152,* 396–411.

Greendale, G. A., Petersen, L., Zibecchi, L., & Ganz, P. A. (2001). Factors related to sexual function in postmenopausal women with a history of breast cancer. *Menopause: The Journal of The North American Menopause Society, 8,* 111–119.

Harmer, V. (2006). The psychological implications of breast cancer. *Practice Nurse, 32*(6), 44–49.

Hartman, S. (2004). Reading the scar in breast cancer poetry. *Feminist Studies, 30,* 155–177.

Henson, H. K., (2002). Breast cancer and sexuality. *Sexuality and Disability, 20*(4), 261–275.

Heyman, R. E., & Vivian, D. (1997). *RMICS: Rapid Marital Interaction Coding System; Training manual for coders.* Unpublished manuscript, State University of New York at Stony Brook.

Holmberg, S. K., Scott, L. L., Alexy, W., & Fife, B. L. (2001). Relationship issues of women with breast cancer. *Cancer Nursing, 24*(1), 53–60.

Hordern, A. (2000). Intimacy and sexuality for the woman with breast cancer. *Cancer Nursing, 23*, 230-236.

King, M. T., Kenny, P., Shiell, A., Hall, J., & Boyages, J. (2000). Quality of life three months and one year after first treatment for early stage breast cancer: Influence of treatment and patient characteristics. *Quality of Life Research, 9*(7), 789-800.

Kleinman, A. (1988). *The illness narratives: Suffering, healing, and the human condition.* New York: Basic Books.

Knudson-Martin, C. (2003). Gender and biology: A recursive framework for clinical practice. *Journal of Feminist Family Therapy, 15*, 1-21.

Lewis, F. M., & Hammond, M. A. (1992). Psychosocial adjustment of the family to breast cancer: A longitudinal analysis. *Journal of the American Medical Women's Association, 47*(5), 194-200.

Lewis, J., Manne, S. L., DuHamel, K. N., Johnson Vickburg, S. M., Bovbjerg, D. H., Currie, V., et al. (2001). Social support, intrusive thoughts, and quality of life in breast cancer survivors. *Journal of Behavioral Medicine, 24*(3), 231-245.

Maly, R. C., Leake, B., & Silliman, R. A. (2004). Breast cancer treatment in older women: Impact of the patient-physician interaction. *Journal of the American Geriatrics Society, 52*, 1138-1145.

Manne, S. (1998). Cancer in the marital context: A review of the literature. *Cancer Investigation, 16*(3), 188-202.

Manne, S. (1999). Intrusive thoughts and psychological distress among cancer patients: The role of spouse avoidance and criticism. *Journal of Consulting & Clinical Psychology, 67*, 539-546.

Manne, S. L., Alfieri, T., Taylor, K. L., & Dougherty, J. (1999). Spousal negative responses to cancer patients: The role of social restriction, spouse mood, and relationship satisfaction. *Journal of Consulting & Clinical Psychology, 67*, 352-361.

Manne, S., Ostroff, J., Norton, T. R., Fox, K., Goldstein, L., & Grana, G. (2006). Cancerrelated relationship communication in couples coping with early stage breast cancer. *Psycho-Oncology, 15*, 234-247.

Manne, S., Ostroff, J., Rini, C., Fox, K., Goldstein, L., & Grana, G. (2004). The interpersonal process model of intimacy: The role of self-disclosure, partner disclosure, and partner responsiveness in interactions between breast cancer patients and their partners. *Journal of Family Psychology, 18*, 589-99.

Manne, S., Ostroff, J., Winkel, G., Goldstein, L., Fox, K., & Grana, G. (2004). Posttraumatic growth after breast cancer: Patient, partner, and couple perspectives. *Psychosomatic Medicine, 66*, 442-454.

Manne, S., Sherman, M., Ross, S., Ostroff, J., Heyman, R. E., & Fox, K. (2004). Couples' support-related communication, psychological distress, and relationship satisfaction among women with early stage breast cancer. *Journal of Consulting and Clinical Psychology, 72*, 660-670.

Manne, S. L., Taylor, K., Dougherty, W. J., & Kemeny, N. (1997). Supportive and negative responses in the partner relationship: Their association with psychological adjustment among individuals with cancer. *Journal of Behavioral Medicine, 20*,101-125.

Manuel, J. C., Burwell, S. R., Crawford, S. L., Lawrence, R. H., Farmer, D. F., Hege, A., et al. (2007). Younger women's perceptions of coping with breast cancer. *Cancer Nursing, 30*(2), 85-94.

McDaniel, S. H., & Cole-Kelly, K. (2003). Gender, couples and illness: A feminist analysis of medical family therapy. In T. J. Goodrich, & L. Silverstein (Eds.), *Feminist family therapy* (pp. 267-280). Washington, DC: American Psychological Association Publications.

McDaniel, S. H., Hepworth, J., & Doherty, W. J. (1992). *Medical family therapy: A biopsychosocial approach to families with health problems.* New York: Basic Books.

Meyer, B. J., Russo, C., & Talbot, A. (1995). Discourse comprehension and problem solving: decisions about the treatment of breast cancer by women across the life span. *Psychology and Aging, 10*, 84-103.

Mor, V., Malin, M., & Alien, S. (1994). Psychosocial outcomes of breast-conserving surgery versus mastectomy: A meta-analytic review. *Health Psychology, 16*, 284-298.

Nissen, M. J., Swensen, K. K., & Kina, E. A. (2002). Quality of life after postmastectomy breast reconstruction. *Oncology Nursing, 29*, 547-553.

Nixon, A. J., Neuberg, D., Hayes, D. F., Gelman, J. L., Connolly, J. L., Schnitt, S., et al. (1994). Relationship of patient age to pathologic features of the tumor and prognosis for patients with stage I or II breast cancer. *Journal of Clinical Oncology, 12,* 888–894.

Northouse, L. L. (1989). A longitudinal study of the adjustment of patients and husbands to breast cancer. *Oncology Nursing Forum, 16,* 511–516.

Northouse, L. L. (1994). Breast cancer in younger women: Effects on interpersonal and family relations. *Journal of the National Cancer Institute Monographs, 16,* 183–190.

Northouse, L. L., Jeffs, M., Cracchiolo-Caraway, A., Lampman, L., & Dorris, G. (1995). Emotional distress reported by women and husbands prior to breast biopsy. *Nursing Research, 44*(4), 196–201.

Northouse, L. L., & Swain, M. A. (1987). Adjustment of patients and partners to the initial impact of breast cancer. *Nursing Research, 36,* 221–225.

Northouse, L. L., Templin, T., & Mood, D. (2001). Couples' adjustment to breast disease during the first year following diagnosis. *Journal of Behavioral Medicine, 24*(2), 115–136.

Northouse, L. L., Templin, T., Mood, D., & Oberst, M. (1998). Couples' adjustment to breast cancer and benign breast disease: A longitudinal analysis. *Psycho-Oncology, 7,* 37–48.

Northouse, L. L., Tocco, K. M., & West, P. (1997). Coping with a breast biopsy: How healthcare professionals can help women and their husbands. *Oncology Nursing Forum, 24*(3), 473–480.

Northouse, P. G., & Northouse, L. L. (1987). Communication and cancer: Issues confronting patients, health professionals, and family members. *Journal of Psychosocial Oncology, 5*(3), 17–46.

Orgad, S. (2005). The transformative potential of online communication: The case of breast cancer patients' Internet spaces. *Feminist Media Studies, 5,* 141–61.

Peteet, J., & Greenberg, B. (1995). Marital crises in oncology patients: An approach to initial intervention by primary clinicians. *General Hospital Psychiatry, 17,* 201–207.

Petersen, L., Kruczek, T., & Shaffner, A. (2003). Gender roles and the family life cycle: The case of women with cancer. *Journal of Feminist Family Therapy, 15,* 99–119.

Pistrang, N., & Barker, C. (1995). The partner relationship in psychological response to breast cancer. *Social Science Medicine, 40,* 789–797.

Pitts, V. (2004). Illness and Internet empowerment: Writing and reading breast cancer in cyberspace. *Health, 8,* 33–59.

Rabin, C., & Pinto, B. (2006). Cancer-related beliefs and health behavior change among breast cancer survivors and their first-degree relatives. *Psycho-Oncology, 15,* 701–712.

Rabin, C. S., Pinto, B. M., Trunzo, J. J., Frierson, G. M., & Bucknam, L. M. (2006). Physical activity among breast cancer survivors: Regular exercisers vs participants in a physical activity intervention. *Psycho-Oncology, 15,* 344–354.

Rolland, J. S. (1994a). *Families, illness, and disability: An integrative treatment model.* New York: Basic Books.

Rolland, J. S. (1994b). In sickness and in health: The impact of illness on couples' relationships. *Journal of Marital and Family Therapy, 20,* 327–347.

Rowland, J. H., Desmond, K. A., Meyerowitz, B. E., Belin, T. R., Wyatt, G. E., & Ganz, P. A. (2000). Role of breast reconstructive surgery in physical and emotional outcomes among breast cancer survivors. *Journal of the National Cancer Institute, 92,* 1422–1429.

Sabo, D. (1990). Men, death, anxiety and denial: Critical feminist interpretations of adjustment to mastectomy. In E. Clark (Ed.), *Clinical sociological perspectives on loss and illness* (pp. 71–84). Philadelphia: Charles Press.

Schain, W. S., d'Angelo, T. M., Dunn, M. E., Lichter, A. S., & Pierce, L. J. (1994). Mastectomy versus conservative surgery and radiation therapy: Psychosocial consequences. *Cancer, 73,* 1221–1228.

Schover, L. R. (1994). Sexuality and body image in younger women with breast cancer. *Journal of the National Cancer Institute Monographs, 16,* 177–182.

Schover, L. R. (1999). Psychosocial aspects of infertility and decisions about reproduction in young cancer survivors: A review. *Medical and Pediatric Oncology, 33,* 53–59

Scott, D. W. (1983). Anxiety, critical thinking and information processing during and after breast biopsy. *Nursing Research, 32*(1), 24–28.

Seaburn, D. B., Lorenz, A. D., Gunn, Jr., W. B., Gawinski, B. A., & Mauksch, L. B. (2003). *Models of collaboration: A guide for mental health professionals working with health care practitioners.* New York: Basic Books.

Shands, M. E., Lewis, F. M., Sinsheimer, J., & Cochrane, B. B. (2006). Core concerns of couples living with early stage breast cancer. *Psycho-Oncology, 15,* 1055–1064.

Shields, C. G., & Rousseau, S. L. (2004). A pilot study of an intervention for breast cancer survivors and their spouses. *Family Process, 43,* 95–107.

Swanson G. M., & Lin, C. S. (1994). Survival patterns among younger women with breast cancer: The effects of age, race, stage, and treatment. *Journal of the National Cancer Institute, Monographs, 16,* 69–77.

Takayama, T., & Yamazaki, Y. (2004). How breast cancer outpatients perceive mutual participation in patient-physician interactions. *Patient Education and Counseling, 52,* 279–289.

Thomas-MacLean, R. (2004). Memories of treatment: The immediacy of breast cancer. *Qualitative Health Research, 14,* 628–643.

Vess, J. D., Moreland, J. R., & Schwebel A. I. (1985a). An empirical assessment of the effects of cancer on family role functioning. *Journal of Psychosocial Oncology, 3*(1), 1–16.

Vess, J. D., Moreland, J. R., & Schwebel A. I. (1985b). A follow-up study of role functioning and the psychological environment of families of cancer patients. *Journal of Psychosocial Oncology, 3*(2), 1–14.

Vess, J. D., Moreland, J. R., Schwebel, A. I., & Kraut, E. (1988). Psychosocial needs of cancer patients: Learning from patients and their spouses. *Journal of Psychosocial Oncology, 6,* 31–51.

Wagner, C. D., Bigatti, S. M., & Storniolo, A. M. (2006). Quality of life of husbands of women with breast cancer. *Psycho-Oncology, 15,* 109–120.

Walsh, S. R., & Fortner. (2002). Coming full circle: Family therapy and psychiatry reunite in a training program. *Families, Systems, & Health, 20,* 105–111.

Walsh, S. R., Manuel, J., & Avis, N. E. (2005). The impact of breast cancer on younger women's relationships with their partners and children. *Families, Systems, & Health, 23,* 80–93.

Weiss, T. (2004a). Correlates of posttraumatic growth in husbands of breast cancer survivors. *Psycho-Oncology, 13,* 260–268.

Weiss, T. (2004b). Correlates of posttraumatic growth in married breast cancer survivors. *Journal of Social and Clinical Psychology, 23*(5). 733–746.

Wilkinson, S. (2001). Breast cancer: Feminism, representations and resistance—A commentary on Dorothy Broom's "Reading breast cancer." *Health, 5,* 269–277.

Wilmoth, M. C., Coleman, E. A., Smith, S. C., & Davis, C. (2004). Fatigue, weight gain, and altered sexuality in patients with breast cancer: Exploration of a symptom cluster. *Oncology Nursing Forum, 31*(6), 1069–1075.

Wimberly, S. R., Carver, C. S., Laurenceau, J., Harris, S. D., Antoni, M. H. (2005). Perceived partner reactions to diagnosis and treatment of breast cancer: Impact on psychosocial and psychosexual adjustment. *Journal of Consulting and Clinical Psychology, 73*(2), 300–311.

Yurek, D., Farrar, W., & Anderson, B. L. (2000). Breast cancer surgery: Comparing surgical groups and determining individual differences in postoperative sexuality and body change stress. *Journal of Consulting & Clinical Psychology, 68,* 697–709.

Zahlis, E. H., & Shands, M. E. (1991). Breast cancer: Demands of the illness on the patient's partner. *Journal of Psychosocial Oncology, 9*(1), 75–93.

Index

Note: Figures are indicated by *italics*. Tables are indicated by **bold**.

American Cancer Society 20, 59, 104
Årestedt, L. 51
Armer, J. 44
art therapy 53
Ashing-Giwa, K. T. 25, 66
autoethnography 3–18; writing about painting 5–6; writing about riding 5; writing about writing 4–5

Bakewell R. T. 103
Banks, P. J. 100
biopsy 14–15
Bloom, J. R. 100
body image: body consciousness 62; empirical literature on 21, 60; evaluation 21; gender socialization 62; literature review 22; systematic review 21
Boehmer, U. 25, 66
breast cancer 20; biopsychosocial challenges for 22–4, 62–5, **63**, **64**; case study 108, **109**, 110–14; diagnosis 20, 40, 99–100; mortality rates 20; psychosocial impact 98–9; sexual dysfunction 23; survivorship 104–8; theoretical framework for 21–2, 60–2, *61*, *62*; treatment 20, 24–6, 101–4; younger women with 98–114
breast cancer survivors (BCS) 20, 21; clinical interventions 29–34, 70–5; financial instability 22, 63; financial stability 22, 63; protective factors 23, 64; risk 24, 65; therapeutic interventions 40–55
breast reconstruction 28

Canavarro, M. C. 22, 62
cancer: case study 82–4; clinical course of 81; diagnosis 82; gender-role socialization 84–5; patients in general struggle 81–2
Carter, B. 85
Cash, T. F. 21, 60
Centers for Disease Control Prevention 20, 59
Chang, S. 100
cognitive behavioral model 21
Corey, G. 26, 67

Danhauer, S. 52
Diallo, A. 44
discrimination 9–11, *10*

endometrial cancer, diagnosis and prognosis 7–9, *8*
ethnography 3

Fallin-Bennett, K. 11
feminist therapy 26, 41; breast reconstruction 28, 68–9; child-bearers 27, 68; consciousness raising 31–2, 72; demographic diversity 28, 69; empowerment through photovoice 32–3, 73–4; experiences and perspectives 28, 69; future research 34–5, 75–6; gender role analysis 29–30, 70–1; gender role intervention 30–1, 71; imperfect bodies 27, 68; lack of autonomy 29, 70; limitations 34–5, 75–6; power analysis 31, 71–2; practical implications 34, 75; psychological issues 26, 67; reframing and relabeling 32, 72–3; self-advocacy and treatment navigation 33, 74; social change 32, 73; sociopolitical aspects 33–4; survival rates 28–9, 69–70; treatment disparities 28–9, 65–7, 69–70; Western culture 26–7, 67–8
feminist-informed medical family therapists (FIMedFTs) 106–8, *107*; accept unacceptable feelings 110–11; biological dimension 112; case study 108; facilitate open communication 113–14; gender and power 112–13; increase agency, in patient and partner 111–12; normalize developmental issues 113; open-door policy 114; respect defenses and work through blame 110–11; solicit the illness story 108, **109**, 110
Fingeret, M. C. 21, 60
Frank, A. W. 108, 110
Fritz, H. L. 84

gender role. *see also* feminist therapy: analysis 29–30, 70–1; family life cycle 88–95; family systems 85–8; intervention 30–1, 71; socialization 84–5

Hall, C. 7
Hammond, M. A. 90, 91
Harlow, L. L. 94
heart disease 1
Helgeson, V. S. 84
hospitalization 8, 9

illnessn arrative 17

Jacobs, J. 86

Kennedy, V. 49
Kline, R. M. 34, 75
Kübler-Ross, E. 7

lesbians 4
Lewis, F. M. 90, 91
Li, Y. 48
Lloyd-Williams, M. 49

Mackenzie, M. 52
Macy, S. 5
Manne, S. 101
mastectomy 22
McDaniel, S. 42
McGoldrick, M. 85
Meads, C. 25, 66
mindfulness based stress reduction (MBSR) 52
Moore, D. 25, 66
Moreira, H. 22, 62
Moreland, J. R. 101
Muhamad, M. 44
music 54

National Cancer Institute 21, 60
negative body image 21, 60
Ngamkham, S. 52
Northouse, L. L. 47, 99, 100, 103

open-door policy 114
Orgad, S. 103

Patterson, J. M. 86
Pearse, W. 44
Pitts, V. 103, 104
poetry 53

Radina, M. 44
relationship 11–13, *12*

Rezaei, M. 22, 61
roadblocks 29
Rolland, J. 46, 48, 49
Ruddy, N. 42

Schnoll, R. A. 94
Schwebel A. I. 101
self-care 13–14, *14*
Shands, M. E. 104
Sherman, A. C. 85
Simonton, S. 85
Snyder, K. 44
Spence, J. T. 84
Stenberg, U. 47, 48
Stewart, S. L. 100
Subedi, S. 52
Sullivan, G. 4, 5

Tai Chi 52–3
therapeutic interventions, with breast cancer survivors: care giver role strain 47–50; communication skills and strategies 46–7; diagnosis impacts 40; existential concerns, grieving losses, and family self care 50–1; family climate 41–3; future research 54–5; mind body and expressive art interventions 51; practical implications 54; structural and organizational challenges 47–50; support and psychoeducational resources 44–6; therapeutic assistance 41

uterine papillary serous carcinoma (UPSC) 7

Vess, J. D. 101
Volker, D. L. 103

Weingarten and Dulwich Centre Publications 17
Weiss, T. 105
White, C. A. 21, 60

yoga 52
younger women, with breast cancer: diagnosis 99–100; interactions with physicians 100, 105; psychosocial impact 98–9; relationship stressors and partner communication 99–100, 104–5; sexual relationship 100, 105–6; survivorship 104–8; treatment 101–4

Printed in the United States
by Baker & Taylor Publisher Services